THE
BREASTFEEDING
BOOK

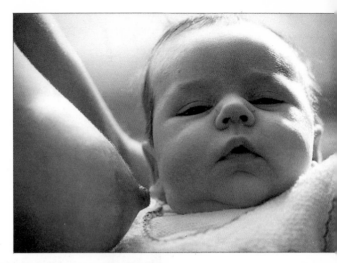

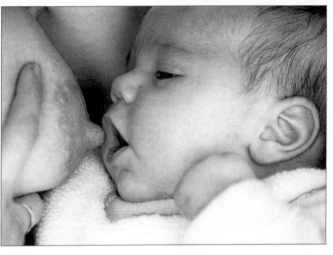

PHOTOGRAPHS

BY

SANDRA

LOUSADA

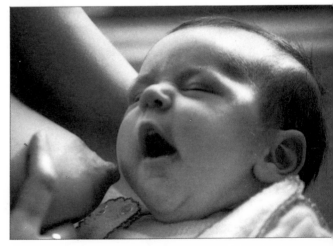

THE
BREASTFEEDING
BOOK

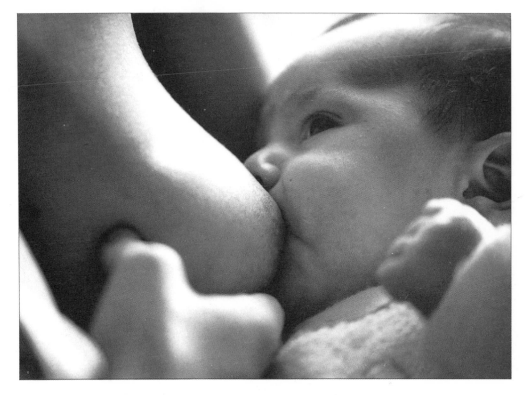

MÁIRE MESSENGER

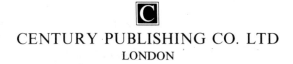

CENTURY PUBLISHING CO. LTD
LONDON

The Breastfeeding Book was conceived, edited
and designed by Frances Lincoln Limited,
91 Clapham High Street, London SW4 7TA

Editor Charyn Jones
Art editor Caroline Hillier
Editorial secretary Gillian Bussell

Managing editor Daphne Wood

Illustrations by Alicia Durdos

Medical Consultants
Dr Michael Hull
Consultant Senior Lecturer
Department of Obstetrics and Gynaecology
Bristol University

Dr Gerald McEnery
Consultant Paediatrician
Whipps Cross Hospital
London

Penelope Samuel SRN SCM RSCN
Breastfeeding tutor
National Childbirth Trust

First published in Great Britain by
Century Publishing Co. Ltd,
76 Old Compton Street,
London W1

ISBN 0 7126 0016 7 (hardback)
ISBN 0 7126 0023 X (paperback)

Filmset by Servis Filmsetting Ltd. Manchester
Photographic services by Robert Horner Photographic Ltd, London
Printed and bound in Italy

Contents

INTRODUCTION

As a breastfeeding counsellor, talking to mothers and fathers in hospitals, clinics and classes, the questions I am most often asked about breastfeeding are: 'How does it work?' and 'What will it be like?'

This book is an attempt to answer those questions as simply, clearly and fully as possible. The information has been drawn from many different sources: medical research; psychological and sociological research; the collective experience and wisdom of the people I have met through the National Childbirth Trust; the written and spoken accounts of many parents; and, very occasionally, from my own experience, where it seemed to fit in with what other people have said. Everybody's experience is different and no one person has all the answers.

I hope that when you have read the book, you will find it easier to make an informed choice, both about how you want to start feeding your baby, and how you want to go on feeding your baby. Much of the information here assumes too that you have not had a baby before because this is the time when books are most useful. Experienced mothers are also catered for, particularly with reference to older children in the breastfeeding family.

Some points of explanation: because most babies in the industrialized world are now born in hospital, you will find more emphasis on the hospital experience than on the fewer feeding problems that arise when a baby is born at home. Throughout the book, the baby is described in alternate chapters as 'he' and 'she'; when the term cows' milk formula or formula is used, I am referring to proprietary brands of baby milk, not pasteurized or untreated milk.

I hope that you will enjoy reading the book – and looking

at it. Breastfeeding information has little attractive, well-designed material to rival the glossy advertisements and brochures of the baby-milk manufacturers. The designer, artist, photographer and editor who have worked on *The Breastfeeding Book* have, I think, redressed some of that balance and also made it easier for you to find the information you want when you are in a hurry or a panic.

I would like to thank especially Charyn Jones and Caroline Hillier for their sensitive and imaginative treatment of the text; Dr Gerald McEnery, Dr Michael Hull and Penelope Samuel SRN SCM for checking the text for medical accuracy. Also Dr Tim David, Booth Hall Children's Hospital, Manchester; Dorothy Francis, Chief Dietitian, Hospital for Sick Children, Great Ormond Street, London; Dr Anne Woollet, Averil Clegg and Sue Vicary of the North East London Polytechnic Psychology Department; Shirley Goodwin, Health Visitor in Ealing, London; Anne Buckley, Molly Ludlam, Valerie Osmotherley, Alison Spiro and Richard and Shirley Seel of the Breastfeeding Promotion Group of the NCT; Rhonda Anderson, NCT Librarian at Epping Forest Branch; all for lending me or directing me to sources of information. Also Gill Salmon, antenatal teacher, and the expectant parents in her NCT classes. Thanks to the many teachers, counsellors, health professionals and, above all, parents and babies I have met through my work with the NCT, who have taught me so much, and not only about breastfeeding. Finally, thank you to my family: John, my husband, and Thomas, Hannah, Huw and Elinor, for their inspiration and help. The book is dedicated to them, with my love.

Máire Messenger

1 *THE DECISION*

If you are pregnant, you have probably been asked how you are going to feed your baby. You may be determined that you are going to breastfeed because you have heard that it is best for the baby. You could, of course, be undecided; you'd like to try breastfeeding but fear that you will be too tied to the baby or that it will be embarrassing and restrict your social life. You may not be in favour of breastfeeding at all, thinking that bottlefeeding is much more convenient and up-to-date for the modern mother – but you want to find out something about breastfeeding, if only to confirm your prejudice.

Whoever you are, and whatever you think, it's very likely that you have been given little information about the different feeding methods. It's possible – as many surveys into attitudes and practices surrounding feeding show – that no-one has discussed feeding with you in any detail; that your breasts have not yet been examined by a doctor or a midwife, and that you have not been given any specific advice about breast care. On the other hand you may have been told many different things about feeding, by all kinds of people, and you have no idea who is right or whom to believe. The information in this chapter assumes that you are interested in doing the best thing for your baby and for yourself and your family – but cannot be absolutely sure exactly what that is.

The case for breastfeeding

Breast milk is the perfect food for human babies. It contains all the proteins, fats, carbohydrates, minerals and vitamins necessary for human growth, in the correct proportions for the human baby. These proportions adjust themselves over time to suit the baby's needs (see page 27).

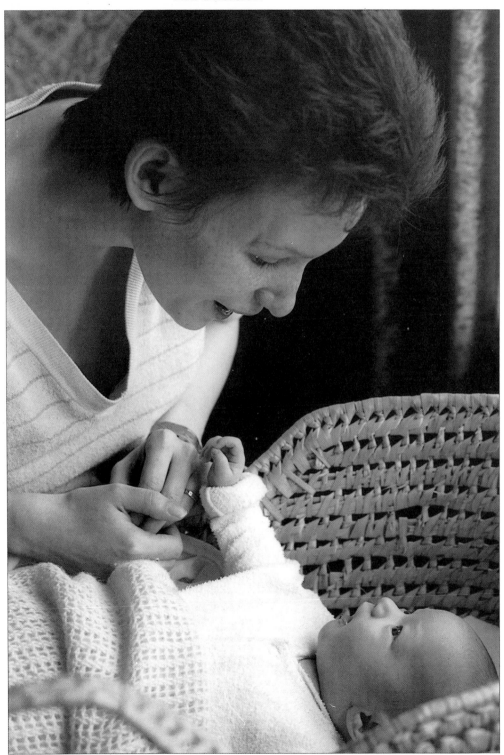

Although this in itself is a strong argument for breastfeeding, there are many other important benefits for both the baby and the parents.

Protection against infection

It used to be thought that breastfed babies suffered less from gastroenteritis, diarrhoea and other dangerous digestive illnesses simply because there was no risk of their being fed from contaminated bottles. In fact, the reduced risk is also because breast milk contains substances that act to protect against infection inside the baby's system and prevent dangerous bacteria from flourishing in the baby's digestive tract. Breast milk also helps to protect babies from respiratory infections and from infectious diseases that the mother has had or has been immunized against.

Protection against allergy

When the newborn infant, with her vulnerable system, is fed on food not designed for her, an allergic reaction can be set up. For example, cows' milk formula contains twice as much protein as human milk and it is 'foreign' protein. The baby's system is vulnerable to proteins that are intended for different species, and it is believed that being given such proteins in the early days of life can set up an allergic reaction, or sensitization, which causes babies to develop unpleasant allergies. People with allergies in their immediate family, such as asthma, eczema or food 'disagreements', are advised to give their babies only breast milk.

Long-term benefits

People who were breastfed as infants are less prone later in life to heart disease and complaints of the digestive tract. Breastfed babies are also less likely to be overweight than bottlefed babies and they are unlikely to suffer from a form of tooth decay in very young children known as bottle caries which is usually the result of feeding the baby with bottles of sweet liquids. Their sucking mechanism too is different from that of bottlefed babies and is harder work. This may contribute to healthy jaw development; certain abnormalities of the mouth and jaw are rarer in children who were breastfed.

Emotional well-being

Many of the claims made by doctors and writers about the superiority of breastfeeding rest on the belief that breastfeeding is better psychologically for the baby. As babies can't tell you (except indirectly) how they feel, this is difficult to prove. But we do know that new babies need physical contact with a warm, caring adult just as much as they need food. During a feed, the breastfed baby, unlike the bottlefed baby, has to be held close to her mother's body or she can't get at the milk.

Sucking

Sucking is one of the great pleasures of a baby's life and the breastfed baby is sucking on a warm, responsive nipple and getting 'messages' back from it (see page 15). Breastfed babies tend to get more sucking experience than bottlefed ones. They are also more likely to be allowed to decide how much sucking they want. Researchers in Cambridge, England, who studied differences between breastfed and bottlefed babies during the first eight days, found that breastfed babies often decided when to stop sucking rather than their mothers making the decision. This was not the case with bottlefeeders.

Feeding and digesting

It has also been suggested that during a feed breastfed babies can recognize changes in the milk composition and are therefore able to control the delivery of the milk by deciding when to stop on one side and start on the other. Another pleasant advantage of breast milk is that it is so easily digested and the bowel movements are always soft.

Bottlefeeding does not give the baby the same range of sensations; she has not the same degree of control over what

Hands, mouth, cheek, skin, heart-beat – all are brought into close contact when a baby nurses at her mother's breast.

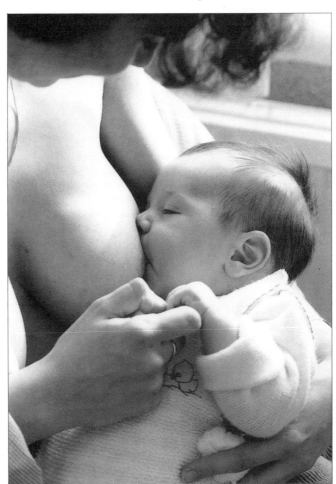

happens. The pleasures of being held by the mother and of having hunger satisfied must be just as great though.

The case for bottlefeeding

There are a few rare cases where breastfeeding may be inadvisable from the start, and there are more frequent cases where, for some reason, the baby is not thriving on breastfeeding, despite the mother's efforts, and has to be given something else.

Drugs

Some women have to take drugs for a particular medical condition and, although many drugs are reasonably safe for the baby because they are either not excreted in the breast milk or because they have no apparent side-effects, some are not. They include: some kinds of barbiturates (for the control of epilepsy, for example); some anti-depressants; some treatments for life-threatening illnesses, such as meningitis, in which case your health obviously takes precedence over the baby's feeding method. If you know you have to take medicines regularly, discuss their possible effects on breastfeeding during your pregnancy with medical staff. There are usually acceptable alternatives for nursing mothers.

Failure to thrive

Sometimes the baby fails to gain weight, and may even lose weight despite your determined efforts to build up your supply. A physical blockage in the baby's stomach, such as pyloric stenosis, could be one reason; this can be easily corrected, once diagnosed, and you can continue breastfeeding. Rarer problems, such as a complete intolerance to lactose (milk sugar), mean that a special substitute food has to be found for the baby.

When breastfeeding has got off to a bad start, for example if the baby had to go into special care, or if you received conflicting advice and tried to take it all, you may never have enough milk to feed the baby fully.

Handicapped babies

Some mentally handicapped babies or those with physical handicaps such as deformity of the jaw or mouth may not be able to suck successfully at the breast, and may need to be bottlefed. Some mothers have succeeded in breastfeeding babies who started life with a handicap (see pages 59–60).

Mother's attitude

If you feel a strong physical revulsion towards breastfeeding, or you are finding it a painful chore, and this feeling persists, the baby will pick up these negative messages and be miserable. Revulsion on your part, like stress, may also interfere with the mechanism that lets the milk flow (the 'let-down reflex', see pages 23–25) and the baby may not get enough. If you really hate the idea of breastfeeding, it will not be right for your baby. Nevertheless, before you opt for

Mother substitutes

**Practical benefits of
breastfeeding for the
parents**
Economy

Nicer nappies

**Benefits of breastfeeding for
the mother**

Convenience

bottlefeeding, it would certainly help to talk these feelings over with a sympathetic person, such as a breastfeeding counsellor or a doctor you trust, and your baby's father.

Bottlefeeding allows the baby to become attached to another person if the mother is not available. It is sometimes said that bottlefeeding is better for involving the father – but there is little research on this. We do know that the father's attitude is important in both the mother's decision to breastfeed and in continuing to do so (see pages 16 and 84).

You do need to eat more to produce the 600 to 800 extra calories used up in milk production daily, but breastfeeding still does not cost as much as buying formula, sterilizing equipment, bottles and so on. You do not need to eat steak and asparagus to get the necessary calories; a few extra nutritious sandwiches can do just as well.

Certainly, if you breastfeed for several months, the economy becomes more apparent since your need for extra food is most urgent in the first weeks after the birth when you are establishing lactation. After that your normal, pre-pregnancy diet, so long as it was adequate, should be enough.

The bowel movements of breastfed babies, which are soft and yellow, do not smell so unpleasant as those of bottlefed babies, which are more like an adult's. Similarly, if the baby brings back any milk by vomiting, this does not smell either. These may seem trivial points, but the physical demands of caring for a new baby can be overwhelming.

In a recent nationwide survey, 80 per cent of mothers who chose breastfeeding said they did so because it was better for the baby's health. Knowing that you are doing the best thing for the baby gives great peace of mind, particularly during epidemics of childhood illnesses.

The next largest group (40 per cent) chose breastfeeding because it was 'convenient' and 23 per cent chose it because it was 'natural'. The convenience of breastfeeding is related to its naturalness. The milk is there, produced by the baby's sucking, always at the right temperature and consistency. There is no need to sterilize bottles and teats, or to mix feeds, or to rush out looking for an open shop because you've run out of formula, or to sit with a screaming baby in a car in a traffic jam. The baby can be tucked under your coat or blouse and fed wherever you happen to be. Breastfeeding is also extremely convenient as a soother of miserable, cross, tired, ill or frightened babies; it is not only a feeding method, it can also be a way of stopping a baby crying, which is a blessing for the majority of us who are deeply disturbed by the sound of a crying baby, particularly at night.

The convenience of breastfeeding becomes more obvious as time goes on, which is a pity, since many mothers give up during the difficulties of the early days and never go on to experience the ease and pleasure of giving a baby a full feed in eight minutes flat, with an arm free for cuddling an older child, or a husband, or holding a book. It also encourages the mother to sit down and relax at regular intervals. Although breastfeeding is time-consuming in the early days, it can save an enormous amount of time later on when the baby has reached some sort of predictable pattern of behaviour, and is feeding less frequently. This predictability is particularly important for working women who continue full breastfeeding.

Hormone activity

The hormones involved in breastfeeding (see pages 22–25) also help the womb to contract quickly back to the size it was before pregnancy and to bring the postnatal discharge to an end. Full breastfeeding (frequent feeding, with no extra bottles) can delay the return of ovulation and menstruation for many months – and this may still be the case even after you introduce solid foods. This is a bonus for women who may have had difficult periods.

Feeding at night need not be tiring and annoying; you can nurse and rest together in the warmth of your bed.

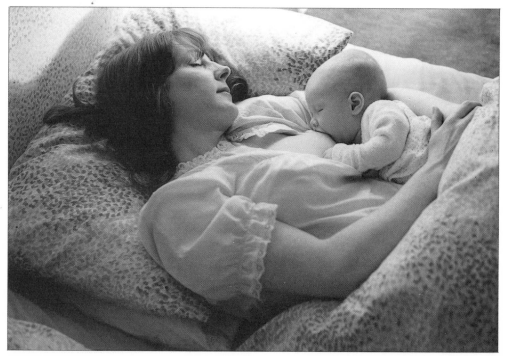

Losing weight

The breastfeeding mother uses up the store of fat that is laid down in pregnancy especially for lactation and so is more likely to get her figure back than the bottlefeeding one. The calories used in milk production may also result in more weight loss – many nursing mothers become slimmer than they were before their pregnancy by the end of breastfeeding. Breastfeeding is not an infallible way of losing weight; some women don't get back to normal until after they've stopped and a woman who was overweight before pregnancy should not rely on lactation to get rid of this extra weight.

Pleasure

Breastfeeding is part of women's sexual functioning and, from the point of view of making a decision to breastfeed or not, the physical, pleasurable intimacy of breastfeeding is a major reason both why women choose to breastfeed – and why they choose *not* to. Some women like the idea of their breasts being used in this way (or at least don't mind), others are embarrassed and ashamed at it. If you are not adamantly opposed to the idea of breastfeeding, it is worth keeping an open mind as your feelings may change after the birth.

Emotional 'feedback'

All through the feed, you are getting feedback from your baby's mouth, from her hands, her body and her eyes. This communicates information to you about how she feels, and what she is doing. Nearly all mothers who continue breastfeeding for some time stress this closeness to the baby as the most satisfying element of breastfeeding. Many nursing mothers are reluctant to stop because it gives them so much pleasure; weaning can be quite a sad experience for them. When you are getting this kind of pleasure, this, in turn, feeds back to the baby. Your smiles, caresses and the relaxation of your body, all help to make the feeding experience more pleasurable for the baby too.

One group of researchers (see page 11) have found that at eight days breastfeeders were more likely than bottlefeeders to kiss, rock and touch their babies while feeding and to talk to the babies between sucking bouts, and this was also true at eight weeks.

Possible drawbacks of breastfeeding for the mother
Physical health

If you suffer from some kind of chronic disease, breastfeeding may be difficult (although, even with serious illnesses such as tuberculosis, it is possible). If you have a regular kidney, lung, or heart complaint or any kind of degenerative or metabolic disease, discuss the possible effects of breastfeeding on your physical health with your doctor, since breastfeeding can be time and energy consuming.

If a woman has had cancer, particularly cancer of the breast, she is usually advised not to breastfeed. It is sometimes claimed that breastfeeding helps to prevent breast cancer – but there is no conclusive evidence about this.

Feeding difficulties

Because the milk is made in the mother's body, and removed from it by a very new person, who may not get the hang of what to do immediately, breastfeeding can cause physical problems (see pages 50–55). None of these, by itself, is insuperable. However, in some mothers, a combination of tiredness, pain, feelings of failure and depression may make breastfeeding just too difficult and bottlefeeding has to be the answer. Support, reassurance and good advice can make such situations less likely.

The father's attitude

The decision about how the baby should be fed should be a joint one between the parents. Many fathers are eager for their babies to be breastfed. If the expectant father is against the idea of breastfeeding, however, you should talk it over with him – and, if possible, get him to discuss it with some other fathers who have babies. It can help for him to see a baby being breastfed and to read about the subject. The problem certainly should not be ignored, particularly if you want to breastfeed. The main thing is that you should agree.

The father may feel that, because you do all the feeding, he has less part to play – in either your life, or the baby's. Such feelings of rejection can upset the early weeks of the baby's life and may even get worse.

Social attitudes

In 1915, a young man called W. N. P. Barbellion noted in his diary (later published) that a woman on a bus, on which he was travelling, tried to breastfeed her screaming baby; when the baby wouldn't take the breast, the woman said she would 'give it to the gentleman opposite'. Barbellion commented matter-of-factly: 'Do I look undernourished?' and passed on to other topics. Despite a revolution in sexual attitudes since the 1960s, attitudes to breastfeeding in public seem to have travelled backwards. Even if you feel no embarrassment about feeding in a public place, it seems from the publicized outcries that occur from time to time that other people do find it embarrassing. When you are breastfeeding in public or at a social gathering, you come to realize that these attitudes are rife, probably because people are just not used to seeing babies being breastfed. A shawl is probably the best solution, though you must try not to let these reactions upset you or your milk production may be affected (see page 24).

Can I do it?

If you are still in doubt about your potential as a breastfeeder, try some of the questions on the opposite page. The answers may help you to sort out your true feelings.

What do I feel about breastfeeding?
How do I feel when I see it done?

How long could I breastfeed for?
Could I see myself feeding a toddler?

What do I feel about bottlefeeding?
How do I feel when I see it done?

Could I see myself feeding with a bottle after the first few weeks or months?

How do I feel about the changes in my breasts during pregnancy?

How does my husband/partner feel about all these things?

If I had feeding problems with my first child, what went wrong?

If feeding went well, will it go so well this time or will my older children be a problem?
What sort of problems might they cause?
Does my husband/partner know about these problems?
What might he do to help with older children?

What people will I have around to help me when the baby comes and how do they feel about breastfeeding?

What did my mother and mother-in-law do?
What do they feel about their feeding experiences?

What have I heard about breastfeeding from other people?
On what was their information based?
Do I trust this information – and if not, who else can I ask that I do trust?

Am I hoping to go back to work/voluntary activities/social life/sport, sooner or later?
How will breastfeeding fit in with this?
How will bottlefeeding fit in with this?
How important are these activities to me?

Do I like to be organized, tidy, predictable?

Am I untidy, disorganized, unpredictable?

Am I organized in some situations, easy going in others – and what are these situations?

You may not be able to give answers to all these questions, and you won't know some of them until you actually have the baby. The only advice an outsider can give is that if you are eager to breastfeed, think in advance about some of the possible effects breastfeeding will have on your life and some of the possible problems. Face, too, the possibility that you may one day end up bottlefeeding (the majority of breast-feeding mothers do, some reluctantly, some with relief) and think constructively about that (see pages 81–82).

If you are eager to bottlefeed and are unconvinced by the health advantages of breastfeeding and the possibilities of enjoyment for the mother, remember that cuddling, caress-ing, holding, playing and caring are what your baby also needs. Being able to 'hand the baby over' may not be an advantage in practice; enjoy your baby in every way possible. And be careful about using the correct formula, making it up properly and sterilization (see page 83).

If you are still undecided – then it is worth giving breastfeeding a try. You can always change to bottlefeeding if you don't like it (whereas you will find it extremely difficult to change from bottle to breast). Just a few days of breastfeeding will give your baby an excellent start in life, and you may discover that breastfeeding *is* right for you.

2 *HOW YOUR BODY MAKES MILK*

Many of our body functions are controlled and influenced by the actions of hormones. A special area in the brain, the hypothalamus, sends substances known as releasing factors through local blood vessels to the pituitary gland, situated just below the brain, which in turn releases the hormones or 'chemical messengers' via the bloodstream to the appropriate part of the body. For example, it is the secretion of the hormone FSH (follicle stimulating hormone) by the hypothalamus that stimulates the ovaries causing oestrogen to rise to such levels in young girls that menstruation begins. Our reproductive processes are dependent on a complex variety of hormones, and lactation is no exception.

The breasts

Human beings are mammals, which means that they make milk for their young. There are all kinds of ways in which different creatures are equipped to produce this milk – from the flat nipple inside the kangaroo's pouch, to the impressive row of teats on the mother pig. The human mother has two mammary glands – her breasts.

In the last half of this century, especially in the developed world, breasts have become more noticeably a way of attracting men, and their main function – feeding – has been lost. Some people now think of breasts as something sexy and erotic and the idea of using them to nourish babies has absurdly come to seem strange and rather indecent. This is a pity, since the pleasurable function of breasts and their useful nourishing function are obviously linked; breastfeeding had to be enjoyable to ensure that human mothers suckled their young and helped them to survive.

How the breasts develop

All newborn infants, both boys and girls, have rudimentary breasts with a nipple and areola. Some babies even

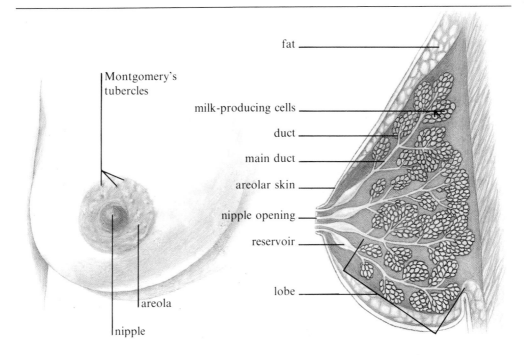

fat

Montgomery's tubercles

milk-producing cells

duct

main duct

areolar skin

nipple opening

reservoir

lobe

areola

nipple

The cross section of each lobe in the breast is often likened to a tree with a trunk (main duct), branches and leaves.

Adolescence

Adulthood

produce a little milk in the first days after birth, due to the fact that the mother's hormones, which have crossed from the placenta, are still circulating in the baby's body. Both sexes are flat-chested until the tenth or eleventh year, when both begin to enlarge slightly. The male breast then stops developing, but the female breast starts to change.

Under the influence of the hormones oestrogen and progesterone, which begin to be produced by the ovaries as adolescence gets under way, the breasts develop from the nipple inwards. First the main milk ducts develop, and then, from these, smaller ducts branch out, ending in clusters of cells called alveoli; these will be the milk-producing cells, but, in adolescence, they are hardly developed. The breast is divided into between 15 and 25 segments, called lobes, each with its own duct system. The ducts all converge on the nipple, widening out just before they get there into small reservoirs, called ampullae, which will later hold milk. From here, the ducts continue to the nipple opening. Around the ducts are layers of fat, which give the breasts their shape. The full adult form is usually reached by the mid-teens. Unless they are very heavy, adolescent breasts do not need support.

The mature breast varies a great deal in size from one woman to another. Size bears no relation to the ability to produce milk; indeed, small breasts lactate very efficiently and very large breasts may make breastfeeding difficult physically. Internally, the milk-producing cells are properly developed; they are surrounded by muscle cells (myoepithelial cells), which have a very important function in breastfeeding (see page 23). Women who do not have babies, or who do not choose to breastfeed, still have all this milk-producing equipment in their breasts.

The nipple

The size of the nipple and its surrounding area, the areola, also bears little relation to successful breastfeeding; the important aspect of the nipple is its protractility – its ability to become erect. In its non-erect state, the nipple looks quite flat; but when a woman is aroused in some way, either by sexual excitement, or by being touched, or by being cold or, of course, by contact with a baby, it stands out. Women whose nipples do not stand out in this way have what is termed flat or inverted nipples (see page 32) and may need extra help with breastfeeding (see page 33).

The nipple has a number of openings, between 15 and 25, depending on the number of lobes and main ducts in the breast, and the milk comes out through them like a fountain. Sometimes, milk will leak out through the openings if the breasts are very full or if the small muscle at the base of the nipple is lax. Again, whether they breastfeed or not, all women have these openings.

The areola has a number of small glands called Montgomery's tubercles, which become larger and more noticeable during pregnancy. They act like sweat glands and produce a fluid which helps to keep the nipple soft and supple. Because of the activity of these glands, some experts say that there is no need to use special creams on the nipples.

Breast sensitivity

The nipple is the most sensitive area of the breast, followed by the areola and then the whole breast area. Some interesting research found that this sensitivity varied according to the menstrual cycle, with a peak just before and during menstruation and another peak in the middle of the cycle. The researchers also found that just before labour the nipple was virtually insensitive to contact, but 24 hours afterwards was more sensitive than ever. This indicates the importance of the nerve endings in the nipple for triggering off milk production. The nipple, by these changes in sensitivity, is clearly prepared for its contact with the baby's mouth and sucking action; the vigorous sucking of the new baby and the heightened sensitivity of the nipple act together to get lactation going (see pages 22–25).

The breast in pregnancy

Great changes can take place in your breasts during pregnancy. Tingling sensations, tenderness, darkening of the areola and increase in size can be the earliest signs of pregnancy. Right from conception, the body is preparing the nourishment for the newborn baby.

The most noticeable change is an increase in size, most of which takes place in the early months. An increase of about two bra sizes is a good indicator that lactation will go well. This is caused by a proliferation of the ducts and milk-producing cells which temporarily (during pregnancy and lactation) replace much of the fat that normally pads out the breast. There is also an increased blood supply to the breasts. All this can make them feel very heavy and it is essential for you to support them with a well-fitting bra (see page 32), for comfort and for the sake of your figure in future.

Breasts sometimes develop stretch marks in pregnancy, as does the skin on the stomach. Not much can be done about them, apart from making sure of a well-supporting bra to try to prevent them. Some women can feel positive discomfort and even pain in their breasts during pregnancy, which may be a nuisance but is not of any serious importance unless the breast seems inflamed. The treatment for engorgement (see pages 50–51), plus relaxation and, if the doctor permits, a mild analgesic, can help to relieve this.

Towards the end of pregnancy (from about the fifth month onwards) colostrum may leak from the nipples. This is the fluid that nourishes the newborn before the milk comes in (see page 26). This secretion is triggered by a hormone from the placenta (placental lactogen) and another from your pituitary gland (prolactin). This is quite normal and nothing to worry about. It is also normal if you *don't* notice any colostrum leaking, so don't worry about that either.

Lactation and after

When your baby is born, you will experience one more really dramatic change when the milk comes into your breasts two or three days after delivery. The breasts become bigger than ever, hard, full and uncomfortable. The change is caused by an increased blood supply to the breasts and the start of full lactation and milk production. The heavy, uncomfortable phase, known as engorgement, usually lasts only 24–48 hours, then the breasts become softer again.

In the first two or three months of lactation your breasts will continue to be bigger than usual and to feel hard and full sometimes, especially if the baby goes for a while without wanting to feed. But, after eight to twelve weeks, they will go back to their normal size and will feel soft, just as they did before pregnancy. Many women take this as a sign that they are no longer producing any milk. On the contrary, the breasts may be producing great amounts of milk but, by this stage, the balance between the baby's needs and the amount of milk produced will be right; hence there will not be the build-up and over-production that can cause fullness and discomfort in the early weeks.

By the end of lactation, especially if it has gone on for many months, or even years, some women find that their breasts are smaller than they were to start with. It can take time for the fat that gave them their original shape to replace the extra milk-producing equipment.

The hormones used in milk production
Prolactin

The most important hormone governing the production of milk is prolactin. It is produced by the pituitary gland in small amounts in non-pregnant women but increases greatly during pregnancy under the stimulus of the increasing amounts of oestrogen produced by the placenta. Prolactin, oestrogen and progesterone, and other hormones, all contribute to the growth of the milk-producing cells in the breast

At the delivery of your baby and of the placenta, the levels of the hormones oestrogen and progesterone drop dramatically. This causes another hormone, prolactin, to be released, which starts the production of milk.

1 The baby's sucking at the breast stimulates the nerve endings in the nipple, which send messages to the brain.

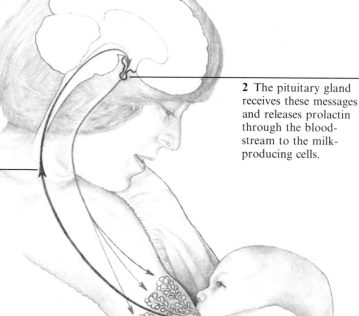

2 The pituitary gland receives these messages and releases prolactin through the blood-stream to the milk-producing cells.

3 Under the influence of prolactin, the milk-producing cells secrete milk in the breast.

during pregnancy. However, milk itself is not produced during pregnancy (apart from a little colostrum – see page 21) because oestrogen and progesterone also inhibit the action of prolactin in stimulating the milk supply. The delivery of the baby and of the placenta removes the inhibiting influence of these hormones, thus allowing prolactin to stimulate production of milk. These hormonal changes will occur after any delivery, even a late miscarriage. Secretion of prolactin is further stimulated in breastfeeding women by a reflex resulting from the baby's sucking at the breast (see page 25).

How prolactin works

Under the influence of prolactin, the milk-producing cells go into action at delivery, although milk production will not be apparent until the second or third day. Then the milk flows out and collects in the ducts, which at first become full and tender. There it will stay, unless it either leaks out or is removed by the nursing baby. The human breast does not have large stores of milk, as some other animals do. It depends for the continuing production of milk on the baby removing the milk at regular intervals so that the milk-producing cells can make more. The baby's sucking at the nipple stimulates its highly sensitive nerve endings to send messages to the brain and, in effect, to 'order' the production of more prolactin. As more prolactin is produced, so the milk-producing cells are stimulated to make more milk. It is thus essential for successful breastfeeding that the baby sucks at the breast at frequent intervals; it is the baby's stimulation of the nipple that keeps the whole milk-production process going and the milk is produced *in accordance with the baby's needs.*

Prolactin production reaches its peak during suckling and is back to its normal level between two and three hours later. Prolactin levels also vary throughout the day, being at their highest in the early hours of the morning.

Prolactin has other important functions, one of which is to suppress ovulation in the nursing mother. Women who breastfeed frequently and unrestrictedly for a long period maintain high prolactin levels and this stops the ovaries producing eggs. The return of menstruation and ovulation can be delayed for months in fully breastfeeding women – one of nature's ways (though not infallible) of arranging child spacing (see page 100).

The let-down reflex

When the baby stimulates the sensitive nerve endings of the nipple, another important hormonal activity is triggered; the pituitary gland produces the hormone oxytocin, which causes the muscle cells round the milk-producing cells and ducts to contract, resulting in the milk being passed on into the reservoirs, thus enabling it to be obtained by the baby. This movement of milk within the breast is called the let-down reflex. The strength of these contractions can be strong; if the baby is removed from the breast just as this let-down is beginning to operate, the milk may spurt out across the room. The activity of oxytocin in getting the milk flowing also causes the womb to contract as in labour, and this is why you will feel afterpains when you first breastfeed.

Hence breastfeeding will help you to regain your flat stomach more quickly; the womb is back to its normal size within about ten days and the discharge from it (lochia) is less prolonged than in the non-breastfeeding mother. Oxytocin, in the form of a nasal spray, may also be used (if available) to get the let-down working if you are having severe problems establishing breastfeeding.

Variations in the let-down

It can take different amounts of time in different women for the let-down reflex to work. For some women, at some times – for example, when they are feeling relaxed and the breasts are full – it can come almost as soon as the baby's mouth touches the nipple. It can even come before that, when the mother hears the baby crying – particularly in a mother who has had some experience of breastfeeding. Other women take longer to let down their milk; it can be a minute or two, or more. This is why it is unwise to restrict sucking time in the early days; there is not enough time to get the let-down going, the milk is not ejected from the cells through the ducts and inadequate stimulation is given for more prolactin, and hence more milk, to be produced.

Let-down failure

A failure of the let-down reflex is probably the most common reason for women not producing enough milk initially. Babies can get some milk – about a third of the feed – by pressing their mouths against the reservoirs behind the areola and drawing off the milk that is present there. This milk is called the foremilk and is low in fat content and hence in calories. But unless the let-down reflex is activated, the baby will not get the rest of the feed – the calorie-rich hindmilk – and he will be dissatisfied, will fail to gain weight and may be weaned onto the bottle unnecessarily.

The let-down usually causes a tingling sensation in the breasts and milk will flow quite noticeably from both of them. Some mothers do have let-downs without feeling anything – but if you feel nothing and are not having a spurt of milk from the non-nursing breast, you may be having let-down problems. One reason could be that the baby is not fixed on the nipple properly (see page 43). Another common

The milk will remain in the breast unless a reflex occurs to supply it to the baby.

2 The posterior lobe of the pituitary gland receives these messages and releases oxytocin, which causes the muscle cells surrounding the milk-producing cells and ducts to contract.

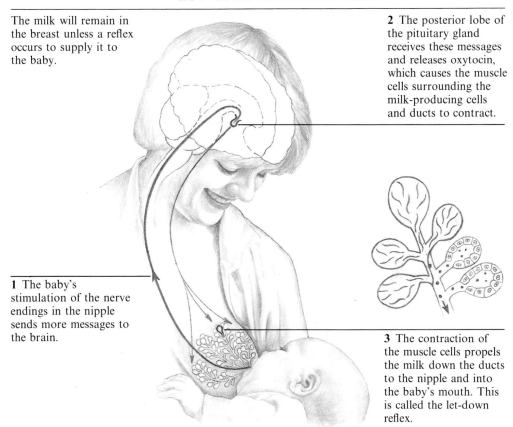

1 The baby's stimulation of the nerve endings in the nipple sends more messages to the brain.

3 The contraction of the muscle cells propels the milk down the ducts to the nipple and into the baby's mouth. This is called the let-down reflex.

reason for let-down failure is psychological: anxiety, stress, pain, embarrassment, homesickness, depression, fear can all interfere with the let-down reflex, presumably by acting through the hypothalamus. Putting the baby to the breast as soon as possible after delivery is important in getting the let-down reflex established.

Solutions to a let-down failure

If it seems that the let-down is not working, various methods can be tried. The most obvious (and difficult) is to remove all sources of stress; it may even mean your early discharge from the hospital if you are worrying about home and are unhappy with the lack of privacy. Conscious efforts to relax, for example using antenatal breathing exercises, or listening to pleasant music, can help.

If your baby is constantly beside you and allowed ready access to the nipple, this will help too. If he doesn't suck well enough to trigger the let-down, gentle massage of the nipple by hand may do the trick. Bathing with hot water and manual expression (see page 34) can work too; once the let-down is going, put the baby to your breast.

Breast milk

We are used to thinking of milk as white, pasteurized, creamy stuff that comes in bottles. The advantage of cows' milk formula is, as so many bottlefeeding mothers assert, that you can see what the baby is getting. This kind of milk is 'real food' and you can measure it. Breast milk is not like that. It *is* real food, of course, but you can't easily measure it or analyse it because it is produced on the spot, in response to the baby's sucking, and it changes in all sorts of ways while it is being produced, even during the course of a feed.

Breast milk is a substance like blood – indeed, it has many of the same constituents as blood and it is manufactured from the mother's blood. The milk produced by the breasts is a continuation of the feeding of the baby while he was in the uterus. If you are doubtful about the existence and reliability of breast milk, it may perhaps help to think of it like that; your baby is nourished efficiently while he is in your womb, without you having to worry about it. The same thing can happen when your baby is born, provided the processes of lactation are understood and trusted, and not frustrated.

Colostrum

This syrupy yellowish substance is the first milk made by the breasts from about the fifth month of pregnancy until about ten days after the birth, by which time it is being mixed with the breast milk proper. The purpose of colostrum appears to be to tide the newborn baby over from his protected life in the womb to the more exposed and potentially dangerous existence outside. Colostrum is different from mature breast milk (see below) in that it has a much higher protein content. The proteins in colostrum contain large amounts of antibodies, which line the baby's intestines, preventing harmful bacteria from entering his bloodstream as well as blocking the absorption into the digestive tract of 'foreign' proteins (see page 10) which might set up an allergic reaction.

With its high protein content, colostrum, even in the small

Comparison of selected components in colostrum, mature human milk and cows' milk (per 100ml/3½oz)

	Colostrum	Human milk	Cows' milk
Energy (kcals)	67	70	66
Fat	3 g	4.2 g	3.7 g
Lactose	5.7 g	7.4 g	4.8 g
Protein	2.3 g	1.07 g	3.5 g
Iron	0.1 mg	0.1 mg	trace
Calcium	48 mg	35 mg	117 mg
Phosphorous	16 mg	15 mg	92 mg
Sodium	50 mg	15 mg	50 mg
Potassium	75 mg	60 mg	140 mg

amounts produced, enables the baby to rest and sleep for long periods in the first days after the birth; this rest is needed by both mother and baby after labour. Feeds become more frequent when the mature breast milk comes in.

Colostrum is lower in sugar (lactose) and in fats generally than milk, so the baby's immature digestive system does not have to struggle with ingesting large amounts of fat at first. It does, however, have a higher cholesterol content than milk, which may be important at this stage for promoting the growth of the nervous system and for helping the body to cope with cholesterol later in life. It also has higher levels of some minerals such as zinc, and is rich in Vitamins A, B_{12} and E. It seems to have a laxative effect, and helps to clear the baby's system of meconium, the black, sticky stools produced by the newborn.

Colostrum is very important for giving the baby a good start. It should not be diluted with water or other feeds – it is all a healthy newborn baby needs; even if you give your baby colostrum and then find difficulty in continuing breastfeeding, you will have given him something valuable that a totally bottlefed baby never receives.

Mature milk

When milk begins to be made in the breasts and 'comes in' on the second to fourth day, it is still mixed with colostrum and looks rich and creamy. By the tenth day the mature milk looks thin and watery by comparison. This change in appearance does reflect a change in composition, which is natural and appropriate to the baby's needs. The basic composition of breast milk varies very little across cultures, with even undernourished women producing milk with virtually its full complement of nutritional ingredients (see below).

Changes over time

During the transitional phase (about the first two weeks), the levels of protein and the immunological proportion of the protein in the milk fall (though the baby is taking in far

Composition of breast milk among mothers worldwide (g/100ml)

The various constituents of breast milk are not substantially influenced by the amount the mother eats or by the quality of her diet, as the analysis of breast milk from mothers in different cultures shows. The quantity of milk may, however, be affected.

	Protein	Fat	Lactose
Australia	1.41	4.95	6.46
England	1.07	4.20	7.40
Egypt	0.93	4.01	6.48
India	1.06	3.34	7.47
Indonesia	1.67	3.30	7.14
New Guinea	1.01	2.36	7.34
Pakistan	0.90	2.73	6.20
South Africa	1.35	3.90	7.10
United States	1.27	4.54	7.10

more food and is therefore taking in plenty of protein anyway). Human babies are slow-growing in comparison with other mammals, including calves, and hence need less body-building protein than young cows do. There is also an increase in the lactose and fat content of the milk. The rate of flow also changes during a feed, faster at first, then forcing the baby to work harder to get at the rich hindmilk, which contains the calories. The flow may also allow for the stomach to empty more gradually, perhaps reducing the chances of colic (see pages 74–75). After four to six months the baby may be getting teeth and developing chewing skills, and other foods gradually replace breast milk as the main souce of nutrition.

The ingredients of mature breast milk

Breast milk contains water, proteins for body building, fats for energy and growth, carbohydrates, also for energy and growth, and vitamins and minerals for the maintenance of health, resistance to infection and the building of strong bones and teeth. As already mentioned, the proportions of these ingredients adjust themselves over time to suit the changing needs of the baby and this cannot happen with an artificially prepared formula.

As we do not yet know *all* the ingredients of breast milk, the artificial formula manufacturers cannot ensure that their formulas contain all the components necessary for healthy feeding and growth, and since breast milk has evolved to suit a human baby's needs, we can be reasonably sure that it has everything in it that this human creature needs, just as a cow's milk is best suited to her calf.

Sources of energy

The fat content of breast milk is higher than that of cows' milk formula and it is also different; it has been suggested that the unsaturated fats found in human milk are important for the growth of the brain and nervous system. As there is no loss of fat in the baby's stools, unlike those of a baby fed on cows' milk formula, we can assume that the baby efficiently uses it all.

Iron

Full-term babies have a store of iron left over from their placental nourishment, which sees them through the first three to four months of life (premature babies are different – see page 58). It is now known that the iron in breast milk, though lower than that in cows' milk formula, is absorbed better.

Vitamins

Breast milk contains all the vitamins a baby needs, so long as the mother is enjoying an adequate, balanced diet, including vitamin-rich foods such as fresh vegetables and fruit. It used to be thought that breast milk was lacking in

Vitamin D, which helps increase calcium absorption and prevents rickets, because this vitamin could not be found in much quantity in analyses of the fat content of human milk. In the early 1970s, it was established that there was plenty of Vitamin D in the *water* content of the milk (where nobody had thought of looking before). Therefore, so long as the mother is getting Vitamin D in her diet (fish oils and animal fats, such as butter) or is exposed to sunlight (a major source of Vitamin D) the baby will get enough; extra vitamin supplements are not usually necessary for breastfed babies, but some doctors may recommend them. Formula milks also contain enough Vitamin D to protect the baby. However, excessive supplements of this vitamin can result in a swing in the other direction and cause harmfully high blood levels of calcium, which is usually seen as a failure of the child to thrive. Therefore, meticulous care should be taken when making up the formula, so that the baby receives the correct proportions of essential nutrients.

Anti-infective properties

The presence of protective antibodies in human milk is possibly the most important single difference between breast milk and cows' milk formulas. Cows' milk, as delivered by the cow to the calf, does have protective substances of its own – but processing destroys them.

The immunoglobulins (*immuno* – immunity to infection; and *globulin* – protein in animal tissue) are very special proteins which carry the antibodies to protect the baby from illnesses against which the mother has built up an immunity. When the baby is older, he can manufacture his own antibodies after immunization or infection. But during these first vulnerable months breast milk protects him, particularly against the dangerous illnesses such as whooping cough, *E. coli* gastroenteritis and influenza. For example, one of these anti-infective proteins – lactoferrin – helps to kill off bacteria by denying them the iron they need for growth. Lactoferrin is destroyed by boiling and processing so bottlefed babies miss out on this advantage.

How much milk?

One of the biggest worries for new mothers is that they will not be able to produce enough milk to nourish their babies. The important thing to remember is that milk in your breast is produced to order by your baby's sucking. If he does not suck at your breast often enough, or if his appetite is partially satisfied with water or cows' milk formula, your breasts will not make enough. It is a supply/demand system, and it is usually interference with the *demand* side of it that causes problems with the *supply*. As your baby grows, and his needs become greater, so your supply will increase.

3 *PREPARING TO BREASTFEED*

Every pregnant woman will experience changes in her breasts, whether she intends to breastfeed or not. For the sake of your own comfort, therefore, and for the sake of your figure in the future, you need to take care of your breasts in pregnancy; you also need to take care of yourself generally. This involves both physical and medical care and getting into a happy and confident frame of mind to welcome the baby.

Care of the breasts

The most important aspect of breast care in pregnancy is giving the breasts good support in the form of a well-fitting bra. Most of the increase in size takes place in the early months and it is essential to wear a comfortable bra in a larger size as it becomes necessary. Some women don't like wearing bras – but the increased weight of the breasts may make them feel uncomfortable and stretch marks may occur if the breasts are not supported. The breasts are also less likely to sag afterwards – and this means that those who like going bra-less will be able to do so when lactation is ended.

Nursing bras

You will need a good bra from around the fifth or sixth month of pregnancy, and if you buy a nursing bra it should last you through the first months of lactation. There are a number of different makes of nursing bra on the market and they usually come in two types: those with a flap that lets down so the baby can have access to the nipple, and those that open fully down the front. Front openers are usually preferable to the flap type, as, when the milk comes in and the breasts are uncomfortably full, the 'frame' of the flap may cut into the breast and cause painful pressure and blockage in the ducts. Cotton, or a cotton-polyester mixture, is also better for support than nylon as this tends to get stretchy after repeated washings.

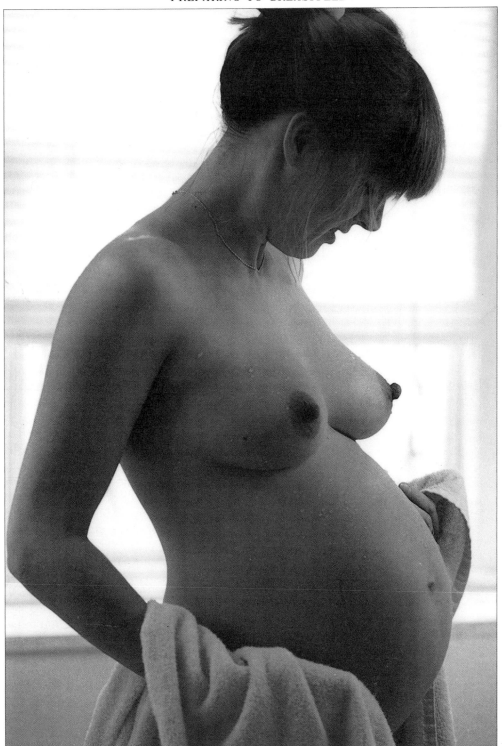

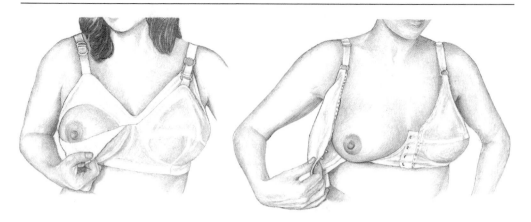

A good supporting bra is essential during pregnancy and lactation. The flap type (left) and the front-opening type (right) both keep the breasts supported, even during feeding.

Babycare shops and chain stores stock bras in a reasonable range of sizes, but if you are an unusual shape – for example if you have a narrow back and very full breasts, or a broad back and small breasts – you may need to be fitted with one of the specialist nursing bras. Some women have great difficulty in finding a comfortable bra that fits and it may be worth contacting one of the breastfeeding organizations (see page 125) if this is your problem.

A well-fitting bra fits closely under the breast and under the arms, without any gaping or cutting into the breast, and it should not flatten the nipples. It should also allow room for the rising bulge of the growing baby. If you are very heavy, you may also need to wear it at night; the so-called 'sleep' bras are not suitable for this purpose, as they don't give much support.

Nipple care

You are likely to receive a great deal of conflicting advice about nipple care, much of it, such as rubbing the nipples with rough towels, extremely off-putting. If you like having your nipples touched, or caressed during lovemaking, this is one of the ideal forms of preparation for breastfeeding. If you don't like having your nipples touched, there is no particular need to do anything to them.

Flat or inverted nipples

Protractility – or the ability of the nipples to stand out – is necessary for successful breastfeeding. To test your nipples for this you can gently squeeze behind them with finger and thumb. If the nipple does not stand out, but stays flat, or even goes inward, you may need extra help. Many flat or inverted nipples automatically correct themselves as pregnancy advances and a vigorously sucking baby can also improve protractility. Mothers who have successfully breastfed one baby rarely have problems with inverted nipples again.

One way of improving flat nipples that is often recommended is to wear breast shields (see below). These are made of glass or plastic and have a hole in the middle; the shield exerts a constant pressure against the areola and the nipple is drawn forward through the hole. They are quite painless and unnoticeable when worn inside the bra. They can be worn from early pregnancy (the problem should be diagnosed at the first hospital antenatal visit at around the 14th week), at first just for an hour or so, and then, towards the end of pregnancy, they can be worn for several hours each day if the mother is comfortable with them.

This exercise is recommended to women with flat or inverted nipples; it involves regular, gentle stretching with the fingers (see below left) which helps to break down the adhesions that occur at the base of flat and inverted nipples. The exercise should be repeated for a couple of minutes each day.

In some women, one nipple may be flat or inverted and the other protruding. You can breastfeed quite successfully from only one breast but every attempt should be made to try to get the baby to nurse on the 'flat' side, if only to prevent

The Hoffman technique

The Hoffman technique involves placing the index fingers on either side of the nipple and gently stretching the areola by drawing them away, then placing them above and below the nipple and doing the same thing.

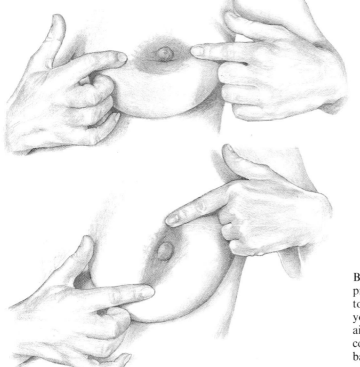

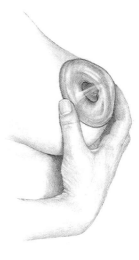

Breast shields are worn during pregnancy and after the birth to improve protractility. If you wear the shield with the airhole uppermost, you can collect leaking milk while the baby is on the other breast.

engagement and discomfort. In a very few women, especially those whose babies, for some reason, do not suck very efficiently, inverted nipples may prevent them from breastfeeding at all. This eventuality has to be borne in mind, but it is still possible for the milk to be expressed and given to the baby in a bottle.

Creams and sprays

Women are often recommended to rub creams or spray aerosols onto their nipples in pregnancy to prepare them for feeding. There is no evidence that this makes any difference. Rubbing a little lanolin or nipple cream into your nipples towards the end of pregnancy may help you to get used to handling this area of your body. Otherwise, the natural oils produced by the Montgomery's tubercles help to prepare the skin quite adequately. Too much soap should not be used on the nipples as it can dry them; splashing with plain water is best. Fresh air and sunshine (in moderation) are much the best treatment for tender nipples.

To massage the breasts before expressing colostrum (or mature milk later on after the baby is born), hold both hands flat against the rib cage on either side of the breast, keeping your arms straight out to the side. Exerting a firm pressure, move your hands lightly inwards towards the areola and nipple.

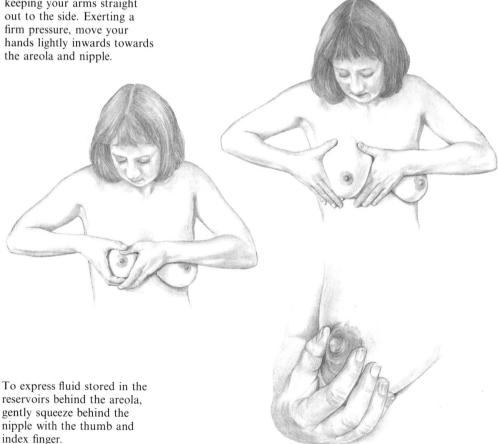

To express fluid stored in the reservoirs behind the areola, gently squeeze behind the nipple with the thumb and index finger.

Expressing colostrum

You may be advised to try to massage your breasts and express colostrum during pregnancy (see opposite). If you notice colostrum leaking, or even if you don't, it can be quite a reassuring exercise to try to express a little in the bath; it helps you to realize that the beginnings of milk production are under way and that everything is working normally. If you can't bear the idea of expressing colostrum, then don't. It will only put you off breastfeeding and not expressing makes no difference to your ability to feed.

Caring for yourself in pregnancy
Nutrition and weight gain

During pregnancy it is important that you take special care of yourself and seek good, regular antenatal care.

Opinions vary as to how much weight the pregnant woman should gain in pregnancy. The average gain is about 12 kg (26½ lb), but some obstetricians prefer women to gain less than this and many quite normal and healthy women gain more.

Weight gain in pregnancy is a result of many factors. For example, the blood volume circulating throughout the body can increase by 30 per cent. After delivery, the fall in hormone levels causes this volume to return to normal.

There are also the obvious factors involved in this weight gain such as the weight of the baby, the breasts and the uterus.

About 4 kg (8¾ lb) of this weight is a fat store specifically for lactation; if you do not breastfeed, you may have difficulty losing this extra fat. On the other hand, if you do not lay down extra fat in pregnancy (and this is true of some undernourished women), you can still breastfeed adequately, as research done in the poorer parts of the world has shown (see page 27).

Although you don't need to eat for two, you will be much healthier if you get plenty of iron (liver, green vegetables) and vitamin-rich foods (fruit, nuts, fish oils) and a reasonable amount of protein (meat, fish, dairy products) and carbohydrates (bread, rice, potatoes). Sweet and starchy

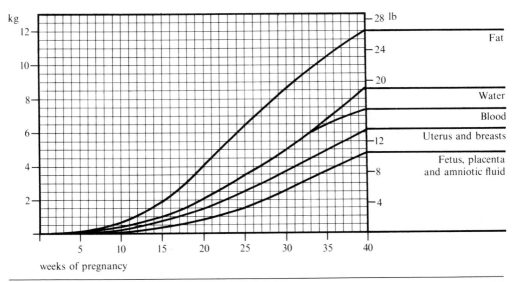

weeks of pregnancy

foods are often frowned upon, particularly in pregnancy, because they can lead to excess weight and its attendant risks of toxaemia (swelling of fingers and ankles, caused by excess of fluid), high blood-pressure and exhaustion. However, in the early months, when you may be suffering from nausea, a sandwich, some biscuits or a bar of chocolate can give a quick energy boost and help you to feel less queasy.

Good eating habits

A breastfed baby can take 600 to 800 calories a day from her mother through her milk. This means you need to eat well regularly when you're nursing, even allowing for the fact that some of those calories will come from the fat store. The ideal time to get into the habit of feeding yourself properly is during pregnancy. There is no need to cook large and elaborate meals; the main thing is to eat regularly at intervals throughout the day.

What to buy in advance

It is a good idea in the last weeks of pregnancy to start stocking up on foods that are simple to prepare afterwards when you come home with the baby. If you have a freezer this is easy to do as you can stock it with ready-made meals. Cans and frozen foods can tide you over the first hectic weeks – so long as they are supplemented with nourishing, *real* convenience foods, such as wholemeal bread, cheese and fresh fruit and vegetables. If you have a lump sum to spare, or generous relatives who want to buy you something, this is the ideal time to invest in labour-saving devices such as an automatic washing machine, tumble dryer or food blender. One baby can generate an astonishing amount of work.

Feeding equipment

Mothers who intend to breastfeed are often uncertain about whether they should have bottles and sterilizing equipment in the house. A reasonable compromise is to have one or two small bottles and teats for occasions when you might want to express your milk and go out, and some chemical sterilizer. There is no need to buy a special sterilizing unit: a covered glass casserole dish, or a plastic freezer container will do just as well. If you use breast or nipple shields (for sore nipples), these will need to be sterilized after use, so sterilizing fluids are useful. But if you don't have any, immersing the equipment in a saucepan of water and boiling for five minutes is just as good in an emergency. There is no point in buying packets of formula as these have a limited life and should not be kept for long, once opened. Formula should be acquired and given to the baby on medical advice only. Beware of free samples handed out in hospitals and clinics. They are not medically necessary; they are simply a form of commercial promotion.

Nursing equipment

Breastfeeding is ideally a simple, natural process requiring only a baby and a willing mother to make it work efficiently. However, one useful gadget, if you need to express for any reason and you find expressing difficult, is a hand pump (see page 73). There are a number of these on the market, and they can be a useful investment for the working mother. The hand pumps that work on the syringe principle are the most efficient. Milk often leaks from the breasts in the early days and a box of disposable nursing breast pads (usually layers of cotton padding between gauze) should be bought before the birth. Large tissues are useful too. A glass or plastic breast shield, such as those used to correct inverted nipples, is useful for catching drips from the breast; the milk can be saved in the refrigerator or freezer. All these things are available from pharmacies or babycare shops.

Clothes

You will need at least three good nursing bras and three nightdresses that open or let down for breastfeeding. Separates are the easiest clothes to wear for nursing as the baby can be tucked underneath them. However, you will probably still have to wear some of your pregnancy clothes after the baby is born until you have got your figure back. It takes six weeks for the pelvic ligaments to firm up – so it's not all extra weight.

Practical considerations
Hospital practices

If you are having your first baby and you intend to breastfeed, it will make your path much smoother if you do everything you can to find out about hospital attitudes to and practices regarding breastfeeding and to discuss your wishes with the staff. If you have a choice of hospital, the hospital's attitude to feeding should be a major factor in your choice. A sizeable group of women abandon breastfeeding before they come out of the hospital so it is obviously wise to investigate any possible problems.

You can, of course, also get information about hospitals from other mothers who have been in them but this information may well be out-of-date and influenced by their own experiences. It is much better if you can build up a good, trusting relationship with the hospital staff directly. Use the questions overleaf as a guide when you pay your first visit to the hospital. If the answers to the questions you ask are all favourable, you should feel encouraged about the hospital. Perhaps even more important, though, is the attitude of the staff to you when you ask them. If the doctors and midwives are anxious to reassure you and to give you information, if they recognize quite happily your right to ask, you will be in good hands.

Questions to ask

Can I feed my baby as soon as he or she is born provided all is well?

Can I feed my baby whenever I want to?

Can I have my baby beside me all the time?

Do the hospital staff in the postnatal wards actively encourage breastfeeding?

Are complementary bottles of formula given to breastfed babies only on medical advice?

Are bottles of glucose and water given to breastfed babies only on medical advice?

If my baby needs special care after the birth, will I still be helped to breastfeed?

Does the hospital have an electric breast pump which I can use if necessary?

Is there a breast milk bank?

When am I likely to be discharged from hospital?

If I am out early, who will look after me?

Is there a member of staff with special responsibility for lactation?

Is there a dietitian and can I meet her?

Are there antenatal classes?

Can I see around the labour wards and postnatal unit?

Will I be able to ask any questions or discuss worries with someone in authority?

Does the hospital have any contact with breastfeeding and community groups?

Can my husband or partner, my other children or other special person visit me regularly?

Antenatal classes

Many hospitals arrange antenatal classes where mothers-to-be are taught breathing and relaxation exercises to help with labour. These classes usually include a session on 'parentcraft' for both parents, and breastfeeding will probably be mentioned then. Many health clinics also run such classes. Although these classes may vary in quality – with some topics dealt with rather superficially, primarily because the classes contain large numbers of parents – it is worth going along to them as a way of meeting other expectant parents, and of familiarizing yourself with the hospital's policies. If you would prefer a more in-depth approach, in a small group, which will often include both mothers and fathers at every session, you can attend classes run by one of the childbirth education organizations (see page 125).

If you can't get to classes, it's still worth asking your health visitor or doctor to introduce you to other mothers with young children or to find out about local groups where they can be found: playgroups, mother and toddler clubs, young wives' clubs, adult education classes can all be a way of breaking down the isolation that a new mother can feel when she is first left with the responsibility of caring for a baby. But do make these contacts in pregnancy if you can; it is harder to find the time or the energy afterwards.

Practical help

Try to fix up someone to come and help you with housework, cooking, washing, shopping and so on in the days after the birth – particularly if you're discharged early.

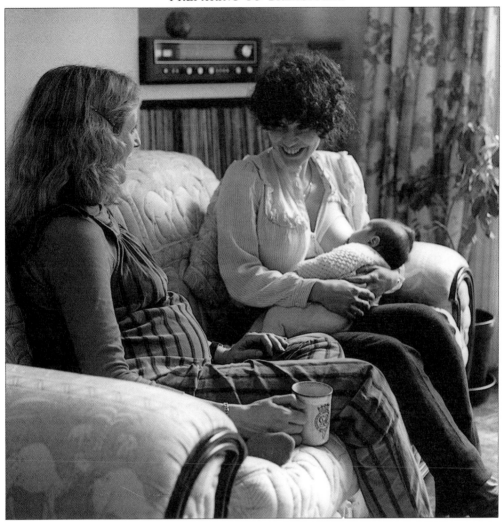

Fathers

*Expectant and new mothers
need the support and friendship
of other nursing mothers.*

If you can't book up a helpful relative and your husband can't get any time off work, ask your health visitor or social services office about the possibility of getting a home help.

Most of the information in this section is also of concern to the baby's father. Going to classes, acquiring information, reading, talking, arranging for practical help, deciding what to spend money on, will be much more valuable as a shared exercise. The idea that mothers need support, help and advice in pregnancy is now generally accepted; but fathers need it too. Being informed and getting together with other parents in the same position is as essential for fathers as it is for mothers – and the best preparation for the shared task of bringing up the children when they arrive.

4 *THE ARRIVAL*

The birth
The importance of early
suckling

There are a number of reasons why putting your baby to the breast as soon as he is born (if both you and your baby are fit and well) is valuable. In the first place, suckling stimulates production of oxytocin, which causes the womb to contract and helps to expel the placenta. Most mothers are given an injection of ergometrine to make sure the placenta comes away quickly, but if, for any reason, it does not come away, suckling encourages the process.

Secondly, because the sucking instinct is so strong at birth, the earlier your baby is allowed to nurse at the breast, the more likely lactation is to be successful. One study found that early suckling (within an hour of delivery) was even more important than frequent feeding in ensuring prolonged and successful breastfeeding – although the combination of early suckling and frequent feeding was most successful of all. Mothers who feed their babies immediately, and more frequently afterwards, produce more milk for their babies.

The third reason for nursing your baby immediately is that it can help to establish a good relationship between you and your baby. Sucking at the breast is an intimate and close physical activity, which is reassuring for the baby after the stress of the labour, and it helps you to re-unite yourself physically with the child that has just left your body.

If either you or your baby needs urgent medical attention, then everything has to wait. This does not mean that breastfeeding will not be successful. If you have had a Caesarean section with a general anaesthetic you may not see your baby for some time. Similarly, if you are all right, but your baby needs medical attention, he may be taken to a special care nursery, or the intensive care nursery in an emergency and your first contact will be delayed.

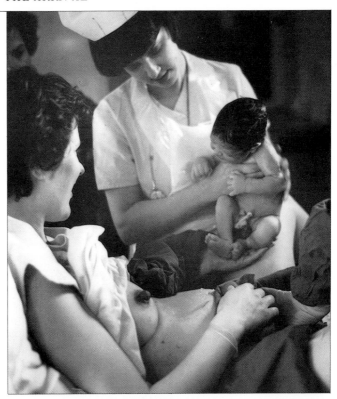

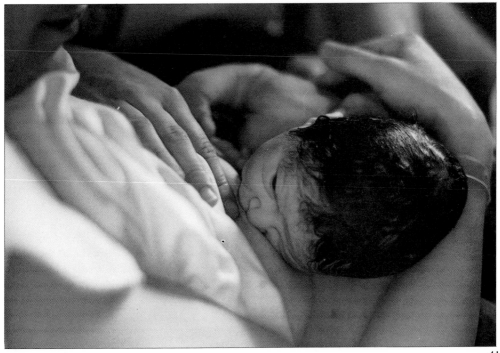

Studies have suggested that the first hour or so after the birth is a sensitive period for the relationship between mother and baby; if you have relaxed and unrestricted contact with each other then, you may, they suggest, get on better later on. If you are separated, anxiety, stress and the actual effects of the illness are almost bound to make the establishment of this relationship more difficult, as well as the establishment of successful breastfeeding. However, if you miss this early contact, do not worry that you can never make up for it. Start from the time you first have real contact with the baby and treat that as the 'birth'. Touch him, stroke him, look into his eyes, unwrap him, hold him close to you and give him time to adjust and learn about being with you. Then you can try that first feed, remembering that he may not get the idea immediately and will need practice.

Effects of the birth process

The early experience of feeding will be happier if both you and your baby are alert and well. This will be the case after a quick uncomplicated delivery, in which you have not been given a lot of drugs, and neither you nor your baby has needed medical assistance in the form of surgery, induction, forceps or vacuum extraction. However, some hospitals routinely give narcotic pain-relievers to mothers, such as pethidine; epidural anaesthesia, which numbs you below the waist; accelerated labour using a synthetic oxytocin drip; and episiotomy, a cut in the vaginal opening to prevent tearing when the baby's head is born. The incidence of inductions, forceps and Caesarean sections has also been increasing. Any one of these can result in you or your baby being drowsy or distressed or both after birth and consequently not very interested in feeding. Drugs in labour can definitely depress the baby's sucking instincts and may make him a sleepy feeder (see pages 54–55).

What the baby can do

A healthy newborn baby has a number of instinctive reflexes that help him to adapt to life outside the womb. He can 'root' around for the nipple and will do so if his cheek is gently touched; he can suck; he can grasp; he will throw up his arms and legs in a defensive movement if he is startled; he can also 'walk' if he is held with his feet touching a flat surface.

He can also cry, and this is often his main means of communication. It is a much less necessary means of communication than many people imagine. If the baby is kept physically close to you, you can tell from his rooting, restlessness, eye gaze or hand movements that he will soon want to be fed, or be picked up, and you can do this before he has to make a lot of noise. Although some babies, no matter how sensitively treated, still need to have a good cry, for many babies there is no need for them to cry at all, unless they are in pain. They do not need to exercise their lungs. Newborn babies are natural learners and begin to adapt themselves to the world amazingly quickly and expertly.

Getting breastfeeding started

The first feed

As soon as your baby is born and has had the mucus removed from his mouth and air passages so that he is breathing well, he can be handed to you and put straight to the breast; some hospitals will do this even before the cord is clamped. Others cut the cord first. The baby need only be wrapped loosely so that he can feel the warmth of your skin next to his. It can be a special moment for the father to take the baby and give him to you and help to get you settled comfortably while the hospital staff attend to you.

How the baby latches on

If you are lying down, the baby can be laid beside you and if you gently stroke his cheek, or touch his cheek with the nipple, he will turn his mouth towards it and try to latch on. The baby may need help to do this properly; gentle support of his head by the father, or midwife, can help to guide him to the correct position. If you are sitting up, you will need to be well supported with pillows, or your partner's arms and body, and a pillow or two on your lap can help to bring the baby nearer to the breast, so that you don't have to support all his weight in your arms.

When the baby latches onto the breast properly (below), he draws the nipple well back into his mouth and 'milks' it with his tongue underneath it. His mouth should be pressing against the areola, not biting on the nipple (below right).

The baby gets the milk (at this stage the high-protein colostrum) by pressing his mouth against the milk reservoirs (see page 19) behind the areola, drawing the nipple back into his mouth against the hard palate and stroking the nipple with his tongue. To get into this position, he needs to be held close to the breast, with his chin against it and his tongue

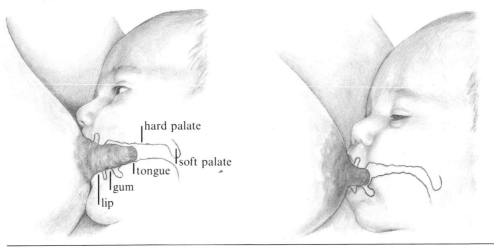

hard palate

soft palate

tongue

gum

lip

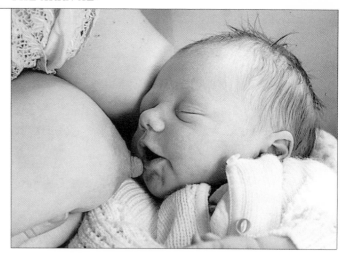

A newborn baby, like other baby mammals, instinctively wants to suck his mother's nipple – but he will need some help from mother and nurse.

Even though he cannot see the nipple, the baby can sense that the breast is near and he will turn his head and root for it.

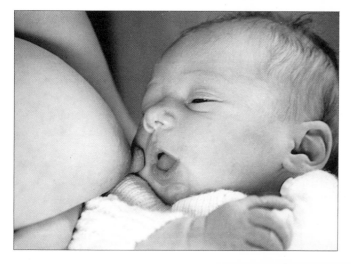

The touch of the nipple on the cheek may encourage him to turn in the right direction and open his mouth.

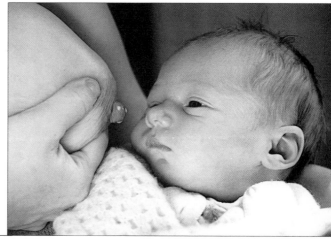

If the baby can't latch on well, or seems reluctant to try nursing, a drop of expressed colostrum on his lips may give him incentive.

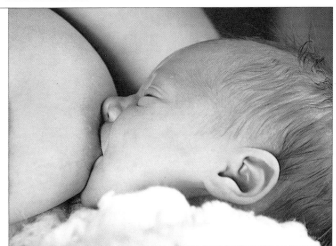

When a new baby is well latched on there should be no gaps between mouth, chin and breast and you will feel that he has the nipple properly in his mouth. You should feel no pain.

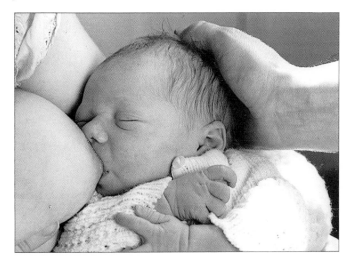

The midwife or father can help to support the baby at the breast while you try to find a comfortable position.

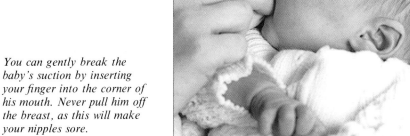

You can gently break the baby's suction by inserting your finger into the corner of his mouth. Never pull him off the breast, as this will make your nipples sore.

under the nipple. Feeding difficulties are often caused by the simple failure to check where the baby's tongue is. The baby does not need to suck on the nipple itself with his mouth, nor should he chew on it with his gums. Correct breastfeeding therefore should not hurt. If it does, the baby is probably not sucking correctly. Ask for the nurse or midwife's help so that you can start again.

Often, at the first feed on the delivery table, the baby will not want to latch on straight away, he may just lick and nuzzle. He should be given as many opportunities as he wants in the next hour or two to have another try. New babies, if they are not drugged or ill, are very alert immediately after the birth and this is the ideal time to get breastfeeding started with a little unhurried practice. Patience and perseverance are essential; there is no need to rush, or force the baby's mouth onto the nipple or fear that he will starve if he is not given a full feed immediately. Nature provides two or three days before the milk fully comes in for mother and baby to adjust to each other.

Getting the baby off the breast

The first feed, during which the baby gets colostrum and sucking practice, will probably be short – perhaps three to four minutes each side (though it can be as long as 20 minutes). The baby may decide to come off the breast himself; if he does not, and you want to take him off so that you can rest, or his father can hold him, you can break the suction by inserting your little finger into his mouth at the corner, or pressing his chin down.

The next feed

Newly delivered mothers are often anxious about when they should next feed their babies. Should you wake him after four hours? Should you let him sleep all night? How will you know what to do? After the delivery, no matter what time of the day or night, mother and baby may want to sleep. Of course, you may be too excited and happy to sleep; the baby too may be alert and wakeful. In such cases, so long as you are in the same room together, you can spend the next few hours lying down, looking at each other, touching and practising nursing. Many women describe these first hours as the most intensely happy experience of their lives.

When to feed

New babies need to be fed when they are hungry and you will know they are hungry by the way they behave. Mothers need to have their breasts emptied when they are full; and you will feel when they are full. Neither mothers nor babies need clocks to tell them when to feed.

The baby will wake when he is hungry and either cry or make rooting movements. He should be put to the breast – the opposite one from the one you started with last time –

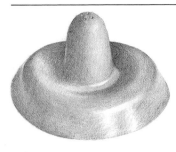

If you have sore or cracked nipples, a rubber nipple shield can be used to protect your nipples when the baby is feeding. It is also used to draw out flat or inverted nipples. Place the shield over your nipple so that the baby can grasp hold of it. His sucking will draw out your nipple and you can then quickly take the nipple shield off and place the baby directly to the breast.

Hospital routines

The start of milk production

and allowed to nurse until he wants to stop. You will feel the milk flowing, you will hear the baby swallowing, you may see milk dribbling out of the side of his mouth. When you stop hearing and seeing these things, the baby has probably emptied the breast.

If you are prone to nipple soreness, or if you are uncomfortably full in the other breast, don't let the baby go on sucking any longer, but switch him over to the other side. If he doesn't want the other side right away, change him, play with him for a while, let him bring up any wind, and then put him to the breast again. He may then sleep for a couple of hours, then want to nurse briefly on both sides and again after a wakeful hour or so. Only after several days will any discernible pattern build up – and it may change week by week. When in doubt, it never does any harm to put the baby to the breast. A good rule in the first few days is if he's awake, feed him.

If you feed in this way, sometimes termed natural feeding, you and your baby will learn to adapt to each other's ways, your baby will get plenty of sucking practice, your breasts will get plenty of stimulation and you will go home from the hospital with a flourishing milk supply. Only when you start up other activities will you need to think about routines.

Many hospitals do not allow breastfeeding to proceed in this easy-going and successful manner. Breastfeeds are given every four hours, with two or three minutes each side for the first day building up gradually to ten minutes each side by the fifth day. If your baby is not satisfied with this (and most babies won't be), you may be advised to give complementary bottles, instead of increasing the number of breastfeeds. This regulated system is based on bottlefeeding and bears virtually no resemblance to the normal behaviour of a breastfed baby and his mother. It will also hinder the onset of milk production, and takes no account of the individual baby. If you are in such a hospital, try to feed your baby whenever either of you wants to, explaining why in a reasonable manner to the medical staff. If this is difficult, remember that you will soon be home and able to do things your own way.

When babies are demand fed, the milk may come in on the second day after delivery and engorgement (see page 21) will be less noticeable. Many newborns don't demand more than three to five feeds in the first two days, so the milk usually comes in on the third or fourth day after delivery. Fortunately this coincides with an increase in demand from the baby; he may want as many as 15 sucklings in 24 hours on the fourth or fifth day. These tend to be quite short and they help

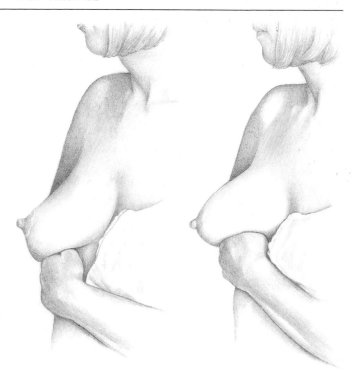

If your breasts are very full before a feed, the soft breast tissue may press against the baby's nose and cause him to panic. Pressing the breast down with a finger to free the baby's nose may block the milk ducts. The best solution is to hold your hand flat against your rib cage beneath the breast (right), then gently raise the breast up a little (far right) so that the nipple is directed down the baby's throat.

This technique is also useful for engorgement, when the nipple may retract if the breast is too swollen.

to relieve engorgement. Both engorgement and number of feeds will subside in the next couple of days until about seven to ten feeds in 24 hours are being given by the end of the first week.

Night feeds

The hospital staff may offer to take the baby out to the nursery for the first three nights so that you can sleep. You can put a card on the crib saying that the baby is breastfed and that you are willing to be woken for feeds – there is the temptation for nursing staff to give the baby a bottle of cows' milk formula. Night feeds are important as if you miss them, supply and demand will not match. It is unrealistic not to wake you as you will be woken at night at home; try to make up for sleep during the day. If you are worried about this, ask to have the baby roomed in with you from the start and you can get used to feeding at night.

Priorities in the first week

Apart from medical care (checks on blood pressure, stitches and so on) you should have four major priorities: rest, a good diet, building up your milk supply, and keeping happy through close contact with your baby and with others who care about you.

Rest

Whenever there is a lull in the day's activities, you should resist the temptation to *do* something and take a nap.

Diet

You will almost certainly feel hungrier and thirstier than usual (particularly after nursing) as you use up the extra calories in milk production. If you find that the hospital mealtimes don't coincide with your hunger pangs, ask your visitors to bring in supplies of snacks and drinks.

Building up the supply

Follow the advice on pages 52–55 if you have any specific problems. Refer to the mechanics of milk production on pages 21–24.

Keeping happy

Most mothers experience a feeling of anti-climax and weepiness on the fourth or fifth day after the birth. It is quite normal and should be treated with understanding by husbands and medical staff. It is natural for you to feel anxious at this time. Try to confide these feelings in someone. There's usually at least one experienced mother to whom you can turn for reassurance, or contact a lay counsellor from one of the breastfeeding organizations (see page 125).

The father

It's hard for your partner to be at home on his own while you get to know your baby intimately. But he can do a lot to boost your confidence and support you during the weepy phases. He can also act as a go-between with the medical staff and as a buffer for unnecessary visitors.

Although you are doing all the feeding, he can do the other things that babies enjoy. Don't criticize the way he handles the baby; he will learn by his mistakes, just as you did.

Common problems with breastfeeding

All the problems in the following chart won't happen to you; perhaps none of them will. Grouped together like this they look daunting. However, they represent the inevitable teething troubles of a new physical process. Most of them will have passed or been resolved within a few weeks of birth – so if you want to breastfeed, it is worth continuing. If you really don't want to breastfeed, these problems can be your pretext for giving up and switching to the bottle. Even a small amount of colostrum and breast milk gives your baby a good start (see page 26), so think in this positive way if you abandon breastfeeding after a time.

While you are in hospital you will come into contact with many members of staff from consultants to ward orderlies: they will all have their own views about breastfeeding and these may conflict. Being well informed yourself is the best defence against this problem. If you are worried, ask the paediatrician or the ward sister for authoritative advice. Politely ignore inaccurate or unwanted advice given by other people. Remember, though, that conflicting advice may be different solutions to a problem: one may work for you and another may work for another mother.

Condition	Symptoms	Causes
Engorge-ment	Hard, full breasts; nipple disappearing into the areola, so the baby finds it difficult to grasp; pain in breasts; skin on breasts shiny and hard. Hot, shivery feelings. Usually on the third or fourth day, passes in 48 hours or so.	The beginning of milk production. The baby may not be emptying the breast fully. Problem becomes worse if he cannot grasp the nipple. Greatly increased blood supply to the breasts builds up pressure which causes fluid to leak into the tissues resulting in swelling. The breasts are liable to bruise easily. Women who choose not to breastfeed may also experience this condition.
Flat or inverted nipples	Nipple fails to become erect when stimulated or when baby sucks. Baby unable to grasp nipple properly in his mouth.	The way you are made.
Sore nipples	Pain when baby first starts to feed.	Pressure caused by the power of the baby's suction.
	Pain throughout feed; reddened skin; raised bumps on skin, sometimes with small blood spots inside them; a whitish stripe across the nipple.	Pressure being applied to the same point at every feed. Nipples being washed with soap. Sensitivity to creams and sprays. Nipples wet all the time, perhaps because of soggy breast pads. Baby sucking too long after breast emptied. Baby not grasping the nipple properly.
Cracked nipples	An opening in the skin which may bleed. Traces of blood in the milk. Acute pain which does not pass as baby continues to feed. Most common on the fourth and fifth day.	As for sore nipples, particularly when the baby is not sucking correctly and is 'chewing' on the nipple. Cracks may develop from a wrongly treated sore nipple or they may develop without warning.

Solutions

Demand feed from the start. If the baby doesn't empty the breast but is satisfied, use a pump (see page 73). Gently disperse the swelling with light strokes of the fingers away from the nipple. Try holding the baby under your arm – it will be easier for him to latch on. Tilt the breast with your hand flat against the rib cage (see page 48). Cold compresses can relieve the pressure if used immediately after a feed. They cause the blood vessels to contract. Warm bathing before feeds can soften the breast and help the nipple to stand out.

The hospital may prescribe pain killers. Bottlefeeding mothers may be given bromocriptine to dry up their milk, or they may have their breasts bound and be advised to reduce fluids.

Put the baby to the breast as soon as possible after the birth. Wear plastic or glass breast shields for about 20 minutes before feeds.

A rubber nipple shield may help to draw the nipple out (see page 47). However, it is the skin-to-skin stimulation of the nipple that is most effective.

Some hand and electric pumps are powerful and draw the nipple out. Put the baby to the breast quickly after using the pump.

Express or pump milk to give to the baby in a bottle.

Be reassured; this is a normal sensation of lactation coming from the let-down reflex and increased nipple sensitivity. It will become less noticeable.

Change feeding position at each feed or even during a feed so that pressure is applied to different points on the breast.

No need to wash before and after feeds. Use plain water on the nipple.

Give up all creams and sprays; dry cornflour is soothing.

Keep nipples dry. Expose them to the air as much as possible. A plastic tea strainer (without the handle) worn inside the bra allows air to circulate round the nipple.

Restrict comfort sucking time.

Ensure the baby is properly latched on (see page 43).

This is very painful and most women find it impossible to continue feeding. There may be a risk of infection through the opening, particularly if the baby has thrush in the mouth – white spots which do not wipe away. Thrush must be treated medically. Take the baby off the breast for a few feeds until the skin is healed. The milk can be expressed and fed to the baby by bottle or spoon.

An antiseptic spray on the nipple before the feed can help to prevent infection.

Painting the nipple with either Friar's Balsam mixed with lanolin, or with gentian violet, can provide a healing protective coating. Reintroduce the baby to the breast slowly for only a couple of minutes at first. A nipple shield (see page 47) can protect the skin until it feels better.

Blocked duct	A noticeable tender lump in the breast or areola which looks red and feels sore. It may be accompanied by hot and shivery feelings.	Pressure on the breast, perhaps from a tight bra. You may be holding the baby too tightly against the breasts, or your own arm may be pressing on the side of the breast. Milk builds up because the ducts aren't being emptied properly; this causes the tender lump. Ducts sometimes get blocked during engorgement.
Mastitis: non-infective	Similar to those associated with blocked ducts; flu-type symptoms more obvious.	This mastitis is caused by milk leaking from a blocked duct into the surrounding tissues and bloodstream. This foreign protein in the bloodstream causes the flu symptoms but it does not mean an infection.
Mastitis: infective	Similar to those associated with blocked ducts; flu-type symptoms are more obvious.	The milk does become infected usually by a germ carried in the baby's nose (perhaps from the hospital). Milk must be tested for the presence of this infection.
Breast abscess	Similar to those for blocked ducts and infective mastitis; the lump may not be so tender.	Failure to treat mastitis. Unnecessary weaning following mastitis. Very rare. Do not confuse with blocked ducts.
Apparently insufficient milk	Weight loss, or lack of weight gain in baby. Scanty, dark-green bowel movements; dry or only slightly damp nappies.	Some weight loss (between 6–10 per cent of body weight) is considered normal in newborn babies; this is natural fluid loss following birth. Can take between 2 and 3 weeks to regain it. Regaining birthweight should therefore be regarded as *weight gain*. Truly demand-fed babies may have little weight loss.
	No experience of let-down reflex or milk flow.	Baby not sucking properly or grasping nipple.
		Feed time being restricted to a few minutes. You could also be tense, thus inhibiting the hormonal activity needed to generate milk production.
		Baby being given bottles of formula or water, which weaken the strength of his sucking.
	Fretful, unhappy baby.	Underfeeding. If nappies are dry and stools scanty and greenish, and there is no weight gain, milk may be insufficient. If nappies are wet and stools soft and yellow, seek other causes.
		Baby may be ill or in pain.
		Baby in need of human contact.

Check for tight bras and uncomfortable positions. Feed the baby lying down for a while.

Offer the affected breast first for a few feeds to ensure really strong sucking and drainage of the block. Lean forward over the baby so that gravity operates too.

Gentle massage of the lump towards the nipple, with hot or cold compresses or a warm hot-water bottle to ease the pain.

Give the baby some extra feeds. *Do not stop feeding*, this will make it much worse.

The doctor will prescribe anti-biotics to make sure that no infection develops in the milk, or to treat one that may already be there (infective mastitis see below). Always take the full course, even if the symptoms disappear. All treatments for engorgement (see pages 50–51) and blocked ducts (see above) can help with both forms of mastitis.

If the milk is infected, the baby may have to be taken off the affected breast temporarily and given extra milk if necessary while you build up your supply on the healthy breast.

Rest, take plenty of fluids. Arm swinging exercises will help to increase bloodflow.

Prompt medical attention: anti-biotics, maybe even surgical drainage. The baby will have to be taken off the affected breast. He can feed from the other until treatment is completed.

Not always a problem. The milk supply can be boosted by more frequent feeds for you and the baby. You should eat more from the start; those mothers who increase their calorie intake are more successful breastfeeders.

Complementary bottles will only reduce your supply further.

There may be other causes for the baby's failure to thrive and he should be medically examined.

Test-weighing is not recommended. It causes anxiety and needs to be done over 2 or 3 days to be at all useful.

Check that the baby's tongue is under the nipple and that his mouth is pressing against the areola (see page 43). Put a pillow on your lap to bring the baby closer to the breast.

It can take time to get the let-down going (see page 24). Extend length of feed times on both sides and let the baby decide when he has had enough. If he is sleepy and not a natural sucker, the let-down can be encouraged by warm bathing and massage or by using a pump. If you are tense, make conscious efforts to relax.

Cut out complements and water – they are not necessary for healthy babies.

Increase the number of breastfeeds to boost supply; if the baby is fretful, nursing will soothe him anyway.

You should be eating well and regularly. Check on the let-down reflex.

Seek doctor's advice.

New babies are sensitive to their surroundings. They are at their

Apparently insufficient milk (cont.)	Fretful, unhappy baby (cont.)	
	Your anxiety and that from those around you.	Lack of confidence in and knowledge about the mechanisms of lactation.
		Desire on the part of others to dominate the inexperienced mother.
Leaking	In the first week or so, milk leaking from breasts between feeds, as well as normal let-down from the non-suckled breast during feeding.	Usually an initial imbalance between demand and supply. Rights itself when the breasts learn to make the right amount for the baby.
	Soaking clothes and bed linen.	There may be pressure on the breasts from the way you are sleeping. This happens often at night when the baby is not feeding so frequently and the breasts become overfull.
		Let-down may occur when you hear your baby cry or think about him.
Sleepy baby	Baby not waking for feeds. Not sucking long during feeds before falling asleep.	Sleepy babies can become seriously underweight and will not stimulate their mother's milk properly. Drugs in labour could still be in the baby's system. You could be taking other medicines, such as sleeping tablets.
		Jaundice makes babies sleepy.
		Hospital ward may be too hot.
		The baby may be ill.
Baby refusing to feed or fighting the breast	As soon as the baby gets near the nipple he arches his back, hurls himself away and punches with his fists. Often follows with screams of frustration and hunger.	The baby's nose may be blocked by mucus so he can't breathe during feeding.
		The baby's lip may be blocking his nose or he may be burying his nose in the breast.
		The baby may have had a bad experience of not being able to breathe while nursing and has become conditioned to panic at subsequent feeds.
		The baby may prefer one breast to the other.

most alert and responsive when held nearly upright over the shoulder or on the lap, supported, so that they can see faces.

Some babies can become irritable and over-stimulated by too much contact; they enjoy the peace of their cribs; they may like to be swaddled. Rocking in a crib has worked since time immemorial. Also rhythmic sounds, such as a recording of 'womb noises', can work.

Keep by you a book or leaflet you have found helpful to refer to in moments of doubt. Eat, sleep and relax.

Recognize that the baby belongs to you and your partner, Diplomatically resist efforts to take over his care from you.

Restrict comfort nursing to slow up excess milk production.

Wear glass or plastic shields (see page 33) inside the bra to catch leaks. The milk can then be donated to a milk bank or, when you get home, frozen for future use.

Feed the baby just before going to sleep yourself. Wear disposable bra pads and strong tissues inside the bra; avoid plastic or waterproof backed pads, which keep the nipple wet. Have at least two changes of bra and clean nightgowns with you in hospital.

Pressure with the heel of the hand against the sides of the breast can slow down milk flow if the baby isn't ready to feed.

A new baby of average or above weight should be fed at least 6 times in 24 hours. Smaller babies (under 2.7 kg [6lb]) should be woken at least 8 times in 24 hours.

To keep the baby awake during a feed, unwrap him, cool him down, and hold him as upright as possible. *Persevere*. If he won't feed, try again in half an hour. If he is alert, feed him.

Jaundice and the effects of medicines need special treatment (see page 60).

Open the window.

Ask the doctor to check the baby if he is very sleepy.

Clear the baby's nose: ask medical staff to help. Hold him more upright while feeding.

Check the position of his upper lip. Support the breast from below with your hand flat against your rib cage (see page 48).

Try fooling the baby by getting him to suck on something else – a finger, a teat, or pacifier. Then get him onto the breast. Try different positions.

Something sweet on the nipple, perhaps a few drops of expressed milk, may encourage him to suck. Try feeding him while he is still half asleep, before he realizes what is going on.

Do not panic. This is very distressing for the mother but tension makes the situation worse. Wait until you are both calm rather than try to feed a screaming baby.

Start with the non-preferred side when the baby is hungriest and has more incentive to suck. Don't turn baby around when changing sides; shift him over so that his feet are under your arm.

Special circumstances in hospital
Caesarean birth

Caesarean births will either be planned (elective sections), perhaps because you are very small, or have a medical condition that makes a normal labour difficult or dangerous, or because the baby would be at risk, or they will be performed as an emergency after you have gone into labour.

In the first case, breastfeeding may proceed more easily afterwards because everyone is prepared; the operation may even be performed with an epidural anaesthetic so that you are fully conscious but numb below the waist. If both you and the baby are well, there need be no problems in getting breastfeeding started, although because of your wound, feeding positions will need to be adjusted.

In the second case, labour may have proceeded for a long time and the operation is performed because the baby is in distress. In this case the baby may have to be taken immediately to the special care nursery for examination and treatment. You may be exhausted from the labour and will have been given a general anaesthetic. Even if the baby is well, he will have received some of the anaesthetic given to you. Getting breastfeeding started therefore may not be so easy. Where the baby cannot suck at the breast in the first hours or days, lactation may be delayed.

Breastfeeding is perfectly possible for the Caesar mother; it is the attendant problem of the operation and the reasons it was done that may cause difficulties.

One feeding position to adopt after a Caesarean delivery is to lie on your side, either propping yourself up with your arm or with pillows, and supporting the baby on pillows under the breast.

If you prefer sitting up, place the baby on your lap on a pillow with his feet under your arm.

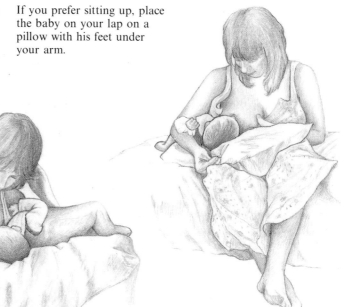

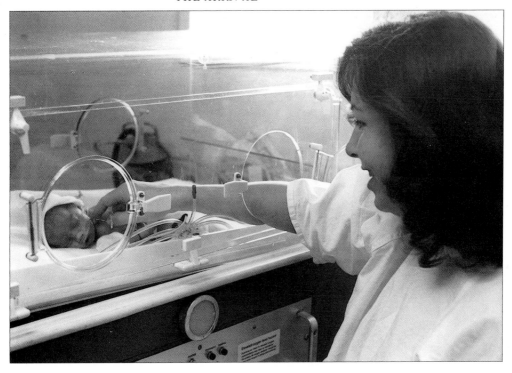

Feeding positions for
Caesareans

The main problem for you is the soreness of your abdominal wound. Holding the baby on your lap may be impossible to start with. You can feed lying on your side, with your shoulder and head supported by pillows, or with your hand supporting your head, and the baby lying under the breast with his feet towards your head. You may need a nurse to help you move the baby to the other side although leaning over a little so that you can offer the baby the other breast minimizes movement. You can also feed sitting up, with the baby lying on a pillow on your lap with his feet under your arm.

You may suffer mild fever – a common occurrence after surgery – and need plenty of fluid and rest. One positive aspect of Caesarean sections is that you always get plenty of bed rest and so can concentrate on feeding your baby for your entire hospital stay.

Premature babies

Even though his life is being sustained with special equipment, your premature baby still needs your loving touch.

When a baby is born before term (40 weeks) there are a number of problems associated with feeding. A very small baby weighing less than 1.8 kg (4 lb), or a baby with breathing difficulties, or both, may need to be kept in an incubator for warmth, observation and monitoring. He may be hooked up to machines, which register his heart rate, and to drips supplying him with intravenous fluids. He may have to be under special lights if he is jaundiced. Lights and buzzers flash on and off to warn staff of changes in his condition. In short, he is put at a distance from you in all kinds of ways and breastfeeding is, at first, impossible.

Even if the baby is not in an incubator, if he is under 36 weeks' gestation, his sucking reflex will be poorly developed and he may be unable to suck at the breast, or even the bottle. His feeds will usually be given by a tube, which passes through his nose into his stomach. Even when the baby is mature enough to be put to the breast, he may tire easily and not stimulate lactation very effectively.

Added to all this, you will almost certainly be feeling anxious about his well-being; you may be in a different part of the hospital; and you may be intimidated by the technicalities and technology involved in your baby's care. None of this makes for successful milk flow.

So how can you manage to breastfeed with so many difficulties? There are a number of factors that can help to motivate you, perhaps more than the mother of a full-term baby. Breast milk is especially valuable for pre-term babies, although very tiny babies under 30 weeks gestation may need special high-energy supplements. Breast milk is easily digested and protects premature babies from infection (see page

Supplying breast milk for a premature baby

When using an electric pump, make sure you are comfortable and try to relax. Use deep-breathing techniques. Apply the cup, which is attached to the beaker, to the breast, turn the machine on and select the required pressure. Your nipple will be rhythmically stretched by the machine and milk should soon start to flow. It should then be transferred from the beaker to a sterile container.

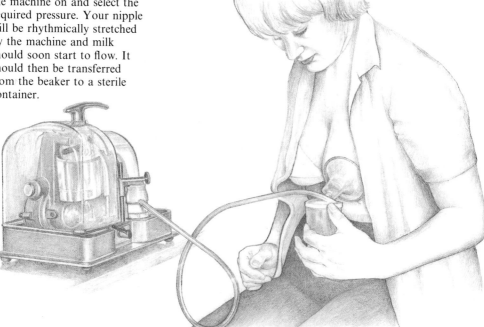

10), plus giving some protection against a particularly dangerous illness sometimes suffered by premature babies – necrotising enterocolitis, a disorder of the intestines. Many hospitals now try to ensure that all pre-term and sick babies are fed on breast milk. Milk expressed, or leaked, by other mothers – both inside and outside the hospital – is kept in a 'bank', bottled in sterile containers and put in a deep freeze.

If you want to express colostrum and milk (see page 34) for your own premature baby, your milk will be given to him and it usually does not need any treatment at all. You will thus be involved in a unique way with your baby's care when you see your expressed milk being fed to him.

Pumping

If you are going to pump your milk for your baby, the electric breast pump makes this task much easier. Most maternity hospitals have them; a minimum use of four or five times a day is recommended. This stimulates the breasts to build up the supply, relieves engorgement and provides precious breast milk for the weak baby.

You should start pumping as soon as possible after birth, so that your baby can get the colostrum right away. Don't worry if the amounts you express by pump seem small in the first few days; premature babies need only very small amounts to start with. When you use the pump, try to relax as much as possible. When your baby is strong and well enough to suck at the breast, he may not get the idea immediately and he may tire quickly. Be patient, and try not to panic. You can continue pumping during this short changeover period to ensure that he has enough milk and that your breasts are stimulated. If you are discharged before him, you can pump milk for him to have when you are not there.

The handicapped child

The birth of a handicapped baby – even when the handicap is correctable, such as a cleft lip and palate – is a shock for the parents. The decision to breastfeed a handicapped baby is a commitment to the baby, particularly on the part of the mother, and she may not be able to make it immediately, so lactation may not proceed easily to start with. Discuss your feelings and possible feeding problems with your doctor.

Cleft lip and palate

Babies whose mouths are not properly formed are going to have obvious difficulties in feeding. They also have the same problems as other babies who require surgery; namely breaks in their feeding patterns while they are operated on and while they recover. Mothers have succeeded in breast-feeding such babies – with great perseverance and commitment. If the stress of getting the baby to suck and the slow weight gain that can result from the interference with the sucking mechanism cause anxiety in the mother and family, then bottlefeeding may be advisable to relieve this stress. A baby with a cleft lip should be held as upright as possible during nursing to stop milk running into his nose and ears.

Mental handicap

There are various forms of mental handicap, some caused by chromosomal abnormality such as Down's syndrome (mongolism), some by brain damage either before or during birth and some by other physical or nervous system defects. A mentally handicapped baby will not be responsive or particularly active and may be sleepy with poor sucking reflexes.

Sometimes mental handicap is associated with physical defects such as intestinal blockage or heart defects. It is possible for a dedicated mother to breastfeed such a baby, with good advice and medical management; he will usually need a much more organized regime, having to be woken for feeds every two or three hours and being fed with great patience and perseverance. There are a number of handicapped children's organizations (see page 125) who can give specific advice and put parents in touch with others in the same position.

Physical handicap

Handicap that does not involve brain damage means that the baby will have the appropriate sucking responses – but the treatment required, for example, extensive surgery in the case of spina bifida babies, usually means difficulty in holding the baby and breaks in the nursing pattern. Obviously, babies who are undergoing surgery need a lot of extra comfort and nursing; you need to be prepared for periods of pumping or expressing your milk when the baby cannot be nursed at the breast. When he is nursed, you may need to feed him lying down or with him lying across you.

Other special circumstances
Jaundice

This is a yellowing of the skin and eyeballs that occurs quite frequently in newborn babies. It is caused by an excess of bilirubin, a waste product that is normally excreted by the liver, but because of the relative immaturity of the liver it is not yet being efficiently excreted. This condition is usually temporary and does not mean that the baby cannot be breastfed. In some cases jaundice is caused by a blood incompatibility between baby and mother and the baby may need a complete exchange transfusion, after which breastfeeding can proceed normally. Phototherapy – placing the baby under a special light panel – also helps to get rid of the bilirubin.

Occasionally jaundice is caused by a hormone in the mother's milk; this is known as 'breast milk jaundice' but, so long as the bilirubin levels are monitored, many doctors feel that to continue breastfeeding is harmless and that this form of jaundice can be tolerated by the baby. Jaundiced babies are sometimes sleepy feeders (see pages 54–55).

Metabolic disorders

Some babies suffer from chemical defects that make it impossible for them to process some of the nutrients in breast milk, which then build up to a poisonous level in the babies' systems. Phenylketonuria (PKU) is an example of such a condition; all babies in Britain are routinely tested for it with a heel-prick blood test about a week after birth. PKU babies cannot process phenylananine, one of the constituents of protein, and have to be fed a special formula that doesn't contain it. However, doctors and nutritionists have managed to devise feeding routines for such babies that include some breast milk in the diet.

Stillbirth

One of the most upsetting of the many distressing aspects of such a tragic event is the fact that the mother's body does not 'know' that there is no baby and generates all the processes of lactation in the normal way. The mother's milk may be dried up by the drug bromocriptine. She should seek expert counselling and be put in touch with a special organization (see page 125).

Multiple births

Twins can be successfully breastfed; the stimulus of two babies sucking produces enough milk for two babies. If you know you are expecting twins, get in touch with the lay breastfeeding organizations (see page 125) and with any twins clubs that may be in your area.

It's easy to nurse twins together. You can combine the regular feeding position for one baby with the other baby facing in the same direction.

When you are feeding lying down, the babies can lie along your body. The lower baby lies in the crook of your arm while the other is supported against your hip.

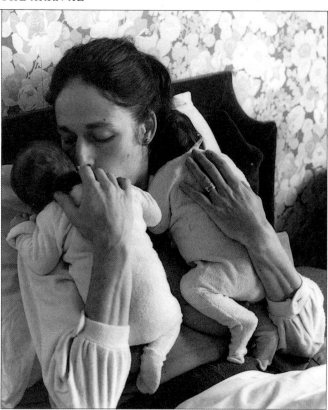

The mother of twins soon becomes practised in handling two babies at once.

When and how to nurse twins

When nursing twins you will be advised to nurse at least three-hourly and some sort of flexible routine may be more practical than full demand feeding in the early days. Twins can either be nursed together, one on each breast, or separately. You may find that you prefer to feed each baby separately to start with, so that you get to know them as individuals. It is usually advisable to feed them one after the other; feed whoever wakes first and then wake the other baby. Many twin babies develop a preference for their 'own' breast and you will probably notice variations in their behaviour with perhaps one being an eager sucker and the other taking his time. Pillows are a great help in nursing twins together. The babies can be laid with their heads on a pillow in your lap and their bodies on side pillows.

Triplets

Mothers have succeeded in giving breast milk to three or more babies, although it obviously takes dedication, as does bottlefeeding in these circumstances. Usually two babies are given a breastfeed and the third has a bottle; the baby having the bottle is different at each feed. The mother may be able to express enough milk to put in the bottle.

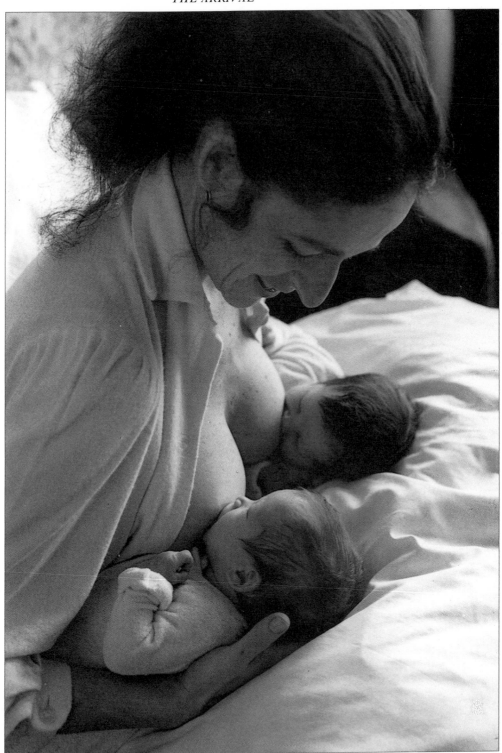

5
COMING HOME

The first days

Coming home from hospital with your new baby is one of the most exciting, but also one of the most nerve-racking events of parenthood. If you are discharged after one or two days, you will need to go back to bed and be based in the bedroom until the health authorities have discharged you. You are both now on your own with the baby – although having a trusted friend, relative or home help around for the next few days can ease the transition.

The first day you are up and about, take things easily. If your partner can arrange to be at home on this day, it will be better for both of you; he can start caring for the baby, and he can do any household tasks and cooking that need to be done. You may feel that you want to get up and about, but don't be tempted. The best thing to do is rest. Visitors should be discouraged on this day too.

Where should the baby sleep?

In the early weeks you may find it more convenient to have the baby sleeping close to you. A crib or cot by the bed means night feeds are less disruptive. Some people recommend having the baby to sleep in the bed with you. If you are happy to do this and your partner is too, it is perfectly safe, and easy for breastfeeding. When the baby stops waking in the night (at any time from a few weeks to several months), you can put her in her own room. There are no hard and fast rules about this – but it is a point on which you may find other people are rather dogmatic. The main thing is to find sleeping arrangements that suit your family.

Some babies and young children continue to wake at night for a year or more; if she does, your baby won't be needing the nutritional value of the milk but is usually looking for comfort. If having her in bed with you is the only way to comfort her, it is a sensible thing to do.

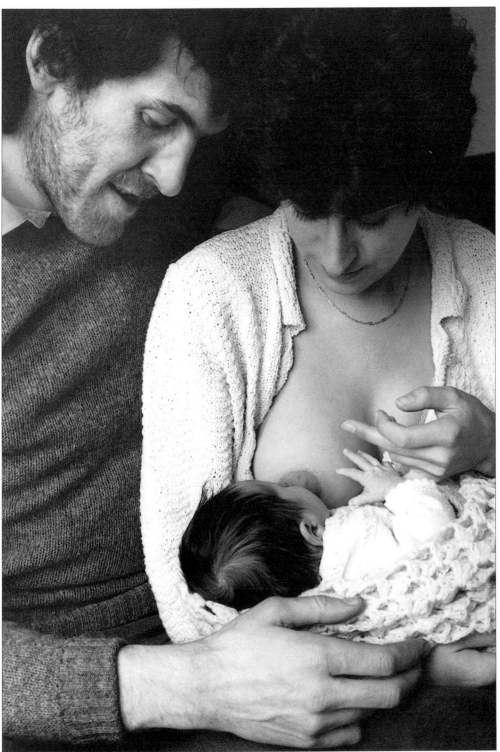

Daytime arrangements

To make your life easier keep the pram or carry cot in the hall or kitchen, so that you can put the baby down to sleep near you if she is fractious during the day. Have a comfortable place (near the telephone) ready for feeding, with plenty of cushions and a book nearby. Remember to get yourself a drink and a snack before starting to nurse. If the weather is bad, you will need to keep the house warm during the first months – about 18–20° C (65–70°F); otherwise the baby may feel the cold and be miserable.

Demand or routine feeding?

If you have been in hospital where demand feeding (see page 47) was the norm, your baby may have found some sort of predictable pattern by the time you are discharged. She may, for example, have a longish sleep in the morning and then want feeding three or four times in the afternoon. She may be a baby who feeds non-stop all evening, then sleeps most of the night, or she may be doing the reverse. Whatever she was doing in hospital, you will probably find that her demands are different when you get home. There may be a complete change of behaviour – and you may interpret this (as nursing mothers often mistakenly do) as a lack of milk. You need

At home, you can organize things so that everything you need is close at hand.

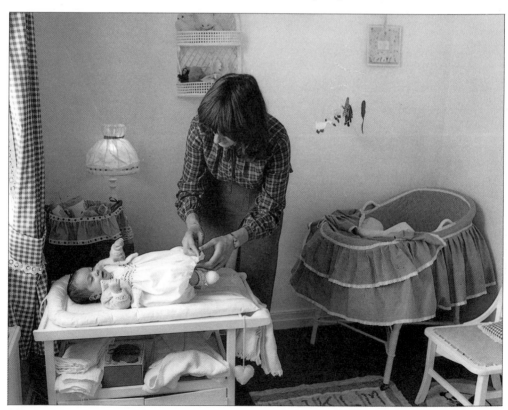

not; babies are sensitive to changes in atmosphere, and in the people around them. Changes in her behaviour are an inevitable part of her growth and development.

If you were in a hospital where your baby was kept to a four-hourly feeding routine and was, perhaps, being given complementary bottles, you will probably find an even more dramatic change in behaviour when you get home. You may now want to start demand feeding and cut out the bottles; be prepared for much more frequent feeds, perhaps every two hours or so until you have completely phased out the complementary feeds. This will help to build up your supply so do not fear that a baby who demands a lot of feeding can't be getting enough milk.

Cutting out bottles

If your baby has come to rely on complementary bottles, your breasts have not been 'told' how much milk your baby needs and are probably not making enough. You may find it difficult to cut out bottles all at once. You can use the chart (below left) as a guide for cutting out bottles gradually, at the same time increasing your own milk supply. Offer the baby the breast first and try giving formula on a spoon. This eliminates the teat, which requires an easier sucking technique and so may make the baby lazy at the breast.

It can take about seven to ten days for the bottles to be cut out altogether and it also takes considerable willpower. If you have become dependent on feeding your baby at set times, with the extra complementary feed to top her up, you may find the adjustment to more frequent and irregular breastfeeding, with no bottles, difficult to make. However, it can be done. The mother who has not been kept to a routine but has learned to breastfeed by getting to know and interpret her baby's behaviour during the first ten days will have a much easier transition to the conditions of the home.

Sample 8-day chart for cutting out complementary bottles

Day	Breast-feeds	Complementary bottles
1	6	4 × 56 ml (2 oz)
2	8–10	3 × 42 ml (1½ oz)
3	8–10	3 × 28 ml (1 oz)
4	9–11	2 × 28 ml (1 oz)
5	9–11	1 × 56 ml (2 oz) (evening)
6	8–10	1 × 42 ml (1½ oz) (evening)
7	8–10	1 × 28 ml (1 oz) (plus water)
8	7–9	none

Conserving energy

If you are giving nine breastfeeds in 24 hours, and each feed lasts, on average, about half an hour, you are spending four and a half hours a day feeding – quite a long time. Many mothers feel that the demands of demand breastfeeding are unrealistic for this reason, although preparation of formula feeds and sterilization of bottlefeeding equipment will be just as time-consuming. Demand feeding works both ways: sometimes *you* can demand a short feed or an earlier one to suit you.

However you feed, your baby is going to take up your time and energy. Both bottlefeeding and breastfeeding mothers will be woken in the night during the first few months so it is sensible to find ways of saving energy.

Some energy-saving suggestions

If your baby is feeding frequently (less than two-hourly), you can keep the feeds short, or you can just offer one side at each feed, if she seems satisfied with it, and if you have something else to do.

Don't bath her every day, just wash her face and bottom.

When you do bath her, to save carrying heavy loads of water, use a baby bath inside the big bath, or put her in the kitchen sink.

Always put a bib or gauze nappy around the baby's neck at feedtime.

Keep a supply of nappies, clothes, bibs and toiletries in the living room as well as in the bedroom; this will reduce the number of journeys you make around the house.

Try to have a nap in the afternoon – even if it's only for 15 minutes.

If you can't, go back to bed after the early morning feed or after breakfast.

Save your energy for times when you know it's going to be needed, for example, when your partner comes home in the evening.

Do something to help yourself relax and enjoy yourself each day; listen to music, watch a film on television, telephone a friend.

And, of course, nurse your baby.

Always breastfeed in a comfortable seat, preferably with your feet up, or lying down (see page 69).

Put the baby in double nappies and one-way liners at night and don't change her in the middle of the night (when she sleeps all night, she's going to go through in the same nappy then).

Obviously, though, if she's moved her bowels or is really soaking, she shouldn't be left uncomfortable.

Use disposable nappies and keep a supply of baby stretch suits and cardigans; this will mean you don't have to launder so often.

Mothers of twins need more extra clothes.

Because breastfed babies' stools are so liquid, if the nappy can't contain them, you may need as many as six changes of garment a day.

If your baby is this frequent, put nappies under her in the crib, so you don't have to wash sheets too.

If you have no help with the housework, do what needs to be done early in the day, including preparation of the evening meal.

Cut down on the ironing.

Use convenience foods, including the 'natural' ones of fresh fruit, bread and cheese.

Accept all offers of help so long as they don't involve you in extra work, like having relatives to stay, who then expect to be entertained.

When visitors come, let them make the tea. If they don't offer to do so, don't give them any.

The right priorities

If you are a competent, well-organized person who has always had a tidy, attractive home and an orderly lifestyle, some of the suggestions in the list above may fill you with horror. Obviously you can't let your standards slide to the point where un-ironed linen and ill-fed husbands are making you so depressed that you can't breastfeed properly anyway. But these early weeks – and these suggestions do apply mainly to the first few weeks – are a time when you have to have the right priorities.

You can't do all the things you did before the baby, and get back to normal after birth and confinement, and breastfeed and get to know your baby and care for her in all the other ways needed. Some things have to come first, and others have to be left for a while. Your baby will be fully

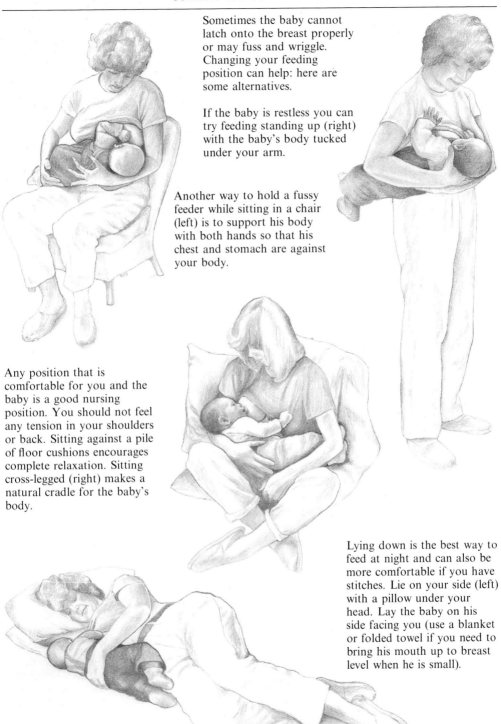

Sometimes the baby cannot latch onto the breast properly or may fuss and wriggle. Changing your feeding position can help: here are some alternatives.

If the baby is restless you can try feeding standing up (right) with the baby's body tucked under your arm.

Another way to hold a fussy feeder while sitting in a chair (left) is to support his body with both hands so that his chest and stomach are against your body.

Any position that is comfortable for you and the baby is a good nursing position. You should not feel any tension in your shoulders or back. Sitting against a pile of floor cushions encourages complete relaxation. Sitting cross-legged (right) makes a natural cradle for the baby's body.

Lying down is the best way to feed at night and can also be more comfortable if you have stitches. Lie on your side (left) with a pillow under your head. Lay the baby on his side facing you (use a blanket or folded towel if you need to bring his mouth up to breast level when he is small).

breastfed (without other foods) for only a few short months. The linen can be ironed any time – and your husband will not die of malnutrition if he has to open a few cans now and then. It can help to write down your daily chores and list them in order of priority. If you can get at least half of them done each day, you're doing well.

If you are a naturally disorganized and haphazard person, these suggestions may seem over-organized. All the same, babies do need things done for them at regular intervals and you will find that they impose an order of their own.

Diet

Breastfeeding requires about 600 to 800 *extra* calories a day over and above what you normally eat to keep yourself well nourished. Some of these calories are required for the actual milk production, the rest are the calorie content of the milk itself. Most of these can be derived from high-energy carbohydrate foods such as bread, cereals, potatoes (which are also sources of vitamins and iron). The extra food thus need not be expensive; only a small amount of extra protein in the form of meat, cheese, eggs or pulses (beans and lentils) is needed. Most people in the developed world already eat more protein than is strictly necessary, so your normal protein intake may well be more than adequate. Drinking cows' milk is also not necessary, as calcium can be derived from green vegetables and cheese.

This is not a time to try to lose weight. Your diet will not affect the quality of your milk but it may affect the quantity and it will certainly affect you. If you are tired and listless, your let-down reflex may not work properly (see page 24). Even then you may not lose weight. Vegetarian (particularly vegan) mothers may need extra supplements of Vitamin B_{12}.

Lactation, produced by frequent sucklings throughout the day, is drawing on your energy reserves and it is therefore important that you distribute these extra calories through the day, so that you do not become overtired as the day wears on. If you are feeling particularly tired towards the evening, note your eating pattern for that day; you may find that your only proper meal is in the evening when you least need it as you will soon be going to bed. Small frequent snacks and three meals a day for the mother are better than one or two snacks during the day and a large meal at night. If you feel hungry during the day, don't feel guilty about eating then; this is what your body is telling you you need. Certain foods – dried or fresh fruit, cheese, honey sandwich, yogurt or milkshake – give a quick energy boost. Don't forget the roughage – wholewheat bread, wholegrain breakfast cereals,

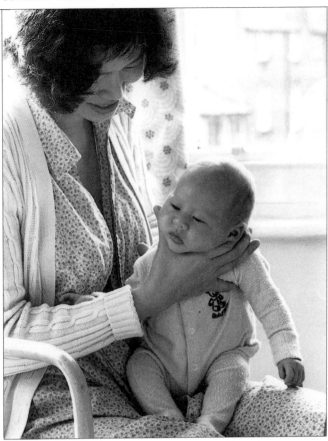

Halfway through a feed, your baby may want to bring some wind up. Hold him upright and gently support his head while you pat his back.

Foods to be avoided

vegetables and fruit. This is particularly important if you have stitches and have a tendency to constipation.

As a general rule, anything that you normally eat should not upset your baby. After all, you have been feeding your baby on your normal diet throughout pregnancy. However, a binge of something you don't normally eat may produce loose, greenish bowel movements and/or fretfulness in the baby the next day. If you notice unusual and irritable behaviour in your baby, think back to what you ate the day before. If there was an excess of something different, try cutting it out and see what happens.

It has been suggested that cows' milk in the mother's diet can result in colicky behaviour in babies (see pages 74–75). If your baby has any of these symptoms, such as constant crying only at certain times of the day or pulling up her legs as if in pain, you can try cutting out dairy products and replacing them with other calcium-containing foods such as extra bread, fish or vegetables and see what happens.

Smoking

A smoky atmosphere is an unhealthy one for a new baby and nicotine does go into the milk. A heavy smoker can produce less milk. However, if you are finding it stressful giving up smoking, the first few weeks after the baby is born are not a good time to put yourself under extra strain. Try to cut down and don't smoke when the baby is around.

Expressing and storing breast milk

There are a number of reasons why you might want to do this. If your baby has been left behind in hospital and you want her to have your milk (see page 58); if you want to go out without the baby and miss a feed or two; for medical reasons, for example resting cracked nipples or relieving engorged breasts; or if you are contributing to a milk bank.

How to collect the milk

Many mothers leak milk during the early weeks; they also let down the milk from both breasts when the baby starts to feed, so it is possible to catch the leakage from the non-suckled breast. The easiest way of collecting these leakages is to wear a glass or plastic breast shield (see page 33). When the shield is full, empty the milk into a sterilized bottle and keep it in the refrigerator, noting the date the milk was collected on the bottle. The leaked milk from five to six feeds can produce about 200 ml (7 fl oz) in one day. If your baby does not use it, or it is not donated to a milk bank, you can freeze it in a sterile plastic container. It may come in useful later – it will keep for up to six months in a freezer and from 48 to 72 hours in a refrigerator. The milk may separate into fat and water layers; just shake it up before use. After about five or six weeks, leaking and copious dripping will decline or even stop altogether. The breasts may also feel softer and flatter. *This does not mean you are not producing enough milk.* So long as your baby is well and gaining weight, it means that supply and demand have dovetailed.

Never let breast milk go to waste – it can be frozen and used for a complement when your baby has a growth spurt later on, or when you go out or go back to work, or to mix with early solids. It does not need boiling. Just use it fresh from the refrigerator – or defrost it when it comes from the freezer and warm it up slightly by placing the bottle in a container full of warm water. Remember that dripped milk has less fat content than milk from the full feed, as most of it will be foremilk, so it may not completely satisfy your baby. Expressed milk, where the breast is fully emptied, will be more like a full feed.

Expressing

Expressing is different from leaking in that you are actually stimulating the breasts to make more milk. You may need to do this if you have missed a feed and are overfull

To use the hand pump, place the plastic cup, which is attached to a feeding bottle (below left), over the breast and hold with one hand (below right). With the other hand, pump with a piston-like action to draw out the nipple and the milk. Remove the pump and the milk is ready in its container to give to the baby.

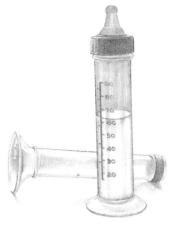

Hand pumps

or if you have cracked nipples. But if you do it in addition to normal feeding, you may have more milk than you need and become uncomfortable. After feeds, or if the baby has not fully emptied one breast, or before you go to bed when the baby is sleeping longer, is the best time for expressing (see page 34).

These are available in a variety of brands. They should be sterilized in cold water sterilizing solution. They are not suitable for use with cracked nipples as they put too much pressure on the painful skin. Hand pumping is quite hard work, but many mothers who can't express find it useful.

For the mother who needs to express all the time, for several days or more, such as the mother whose baby is still in hospital, an electric pump is the best solution (see page 59). These can be hired for use at home.

Voluntary groups

In addition to the professional help available to you in the hospital and after your discharge, there are a number of voluntary self-help groups that have been set up in recent years for mothers at home with babies and young children. Some of these are specifically for breastfeeding mothers: La Leche League was established in the United States and is now worldwide; in Britain there is the National Childbirth Trust; and in Australia there is the Nursing Mothers' Association. (A full list with addresses is given on page 125.) These organizations train mothers, who have successfully breastfed their own babies, to pass on to new mothers the collective experience of nursing women. They can be a valuable source of friendship and moral support.

Common problems

During the first weeks at home while you are learning to understand your baby's needs and demands, the following checklist may help to allay any fears and worries you have about her behaviour and about your reactions to it.

Problem	Symptoms	Causes
Demanding baby	Few breaks between feeds.	Growth spurt, which often occurs around 10–14 days, 3 weeks and 6 weeks. If you check the baby's weight, you will see she has gained a lot at this time.
		Poor let-down reflex, so the baby is not satisfied. Little or no weight gain could suggest this.
		You may be tired and disorientated and see the baby's demands as constant feeding, when in fact they are not.
Constant crying	The baby never seems happy or content.	Hunger.
		Boredom or loneliness.
		Wind or stomach too full.
		Your perception that the baby is constantly crying, which may not be the case.
		The baby may be unwell.
Colic	Baby content for most of day, but has a period of 2–3 hours in afternoon or evening when she screams and cannot be comforted. She may draw up her legs as if in pain; her stomach may feel hard and distended. Usually ends at about 3 months.	Unknown. The mysterious thing about colic is that it occurs only at certain times.
		Cows' milk in your diet.

Solutions
_____

The extra feeding on demand usually produces more milk
within 2 days and the baby becomes more settled. Check your
diet, eat more, and have plenty of rest.

Check the baby's position on the nipple (see page 43).
Consciously try to relax while feeding, and feed the baby when
she is calm. Warm bathing and nipple massage may get the
milk flowing before you put the baby to the nipple. Check other
causes of tension and try to remove them. There is an oxytocin
spray which your doctor may prescribe to help the let-down
reflex work more efficiently.

Make a note of the times you feed the baby. If a pattern
emerges, try to synchronize your other activities with it. You
may find the baby is feeding only 6–8 times in 24 hours which
is quite normal.

Check number of feeds. If only 5–6 in 24 hours, increase to
8–10 if you can manage it. Eat more yourself; and rest.

Carry the baby around in a sling. Play with her, talk to her and
rock her. Accept her need to be sociable.

Hold the baby upright over your shoulder, or on your lap, until
the wind comes up. Apply warmth to her stomach; a warmed
nappy or water bottle wrapped in a nappy. If your baby is
gaining weight, and feels overfull, guide her towards longer
periods between feeds. Let her cry for a while, then go for
walks with the pram, rock or cuddle her to sleep, play with her.

Note the length of time she cries. It may not be as long as you
think. Try to relax. The baby will then relax too. Babies are
often uncannily well behaved when you visit other people. Visit
a friend, it may do you both good.

See your doctor.

Sucking can help. If the baby refuses the breast, or you don't
want to give it, try a pacifier. Keep the baby moving, in a
pram, or a rocking cradle.

Ask others to help you – husbands, relatives, or friends. Try
to keep calm. It is not your fault. Talk to other mothers who
have been through this experience.

The doctor may prescribe a special medicine to relax the
baby's stomach muscles.

Try cutting out all dairy products. Try for at least one week
and see if there is any improvement in the baby's behaviour. If
there is, you will need to continue your dairy-free diet. If there
is no change, return to your normal diet and seek other
solutions.

Sicky baby	Vomiting after nursing.	If the baby is bringing up large amounts of 'curd' and projecting them across the room, she might have a partial obstruction preventing feeds being retained in the stomach. This is known as pyloric stenosis.
	The baby brings up small amounts of milk after feeds.	If the baby is otherwise well, this is usually overflow.
	The baby is sick, and has other symptoms: greenish, smelly bowel movements, a temperature, looks unwell, is listless and miserable.	The baby is almost certainly ill with a stomach infection.

Under-weight baby	The baby is gaining only 30–55 g (1–2 oz) or less a week and is well below her expected weight for age and birthweight.
	    She may be listless and sleep for long periods.
	    Scanty green bowel movements; strong smelling, infrequent urine.
		Illness.
		
		Hunger and underfeeding.
		
		Resuming a contraceptive pill.

Over-weight baby	The baby is fat, well above the expected weight for her age and birthweight. Gains may be 280–450 g (10–16 oz) a week or more.	It is possible for fully breastfed babies to get very fat, though why is not known.
Tiredness and depression in mother	Lack of energy. Inability to organize your life. Indifference to other people. Frequent outbursts of crying for no apparent reason.	Hormonal changes after the birth can result in postpartum depression. Often tiredness is the only reason for irrational outbursts and feelings of inadequacy.
	Lack of interest in the baby; fear that you do not love her or may harm her.	Early problems in the hospital and separation from the baby may have led to anxiety and a poor initial bonding between mother and baby.
		Lack of confidence in mother.
		Difficult baby.

See your doctor, particularly if the baby is not gaining weight. Even if simple surgery is necessary, you can still carry on breastfeeding.

Keep the baby in a bib. Have tissues ready to mop up. It will pass.

See your doctor immediately. Breastfed babies can get gastro-enteritis, though this is rare. Usually breastfeeding is part of the treatment for sick babies, and nursing is a great comfort.

Any vomiting should be reported to your doctor, just to be on the safe side.

The baby should be checked by a doctor in case of any mechanical problem or metabolic illness that prevents the absorption of food.

Try to boost your milk supply (see pages 52–55). A Lact-Aid supplementer (see page 109) may help to keep your supply going if the baby has to have complementary bottles. If supply and weight gain don't improve in 2–3 weeks, complementary bottles will probably be necessary.

If extra feeding doesn't work, you may need to change your contraceptive method (see page 101).

If the baby is having only 5–6 feeds in 24 hours, then do not worry. Weight gain often slows down when other foods are introduced at about 4–6 months. If the baby is feeding very frequently and for long periods, see your doctor and try to reduce the number and length of feeds (if he advises it), but if this makes you and the baby miserable, then don't worry and carry on as before. Accept that your milk is rich in calories and that the baby will slim down when she becomes more active.

Check your eating, sleeping and working patterns. Adjust them if necessary. Sleep when your baby sleeps, get your priorities right. If you feel very depressed, see your doctor. You may be advised to take some medication to get you through this difficult period. Check that it is a drug that is safe for breast-feeding mothers. Psychotherapy or sympathetic counselling can help. See page 125 for helpful organizations. Get in touch with your friends and family. Take your baby to your former place of work and show her off. If you miss your old way of life, make a conscious effort to do something about it. Go out more; tiny babies can be transported easily (see page 110).

Even mothers with no apparent problems find it difficult to love their babies right away. Call your baby by her name, try to see her as a person – kiss, cuddle and hold her. Act loving and the feelings are more likely to come.

Confidence comes with experience: talk to other mothers. You will find that they often had similar feelings.

See advice about crying/demanding babies on the previous page. See your doctor if you are really worried. The fact that you are worried shows that you do care about your baby.

What if you don't succeed?

In a survey done in 1980 of over 5500 mothers and their feeding practices, of the mothers who started breastfeeding (65 per cent), 41 per cent were still breastfeeding at six weeks. Only 5 per cent of the nursing mothers had given up because they had breastfed long enough or as long as planned. Most had given up before they wanted to – in other words, they had failed in what they had set out to do.

The main reasons for giving up in this survey were insufficient milk, then technical problems such as sore nipples. Mothers vary very much. Some manage to feed twins for months, while others find feeding a placid baby every three hours insupportable. Here are some of the breaking points and how to come to terms with them.

Bottlefeeding gives warmth and security too, when it's done with love and enjoyment.

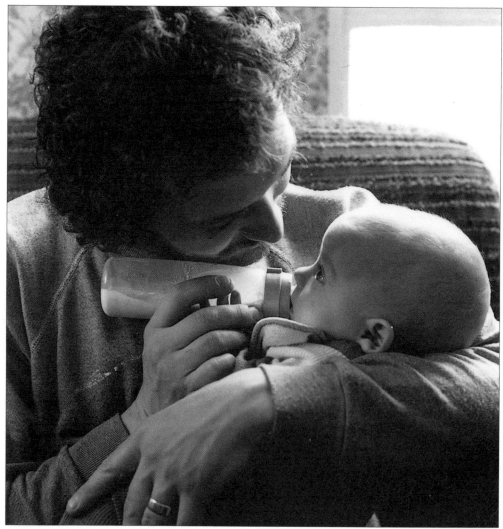

Reasons for giving up	Coming to terms

Failure to thrive in the baby

The baby persistently fails to gain weight and is even losing weight, she needs artificial supplements if she is not to become severely undernourished. Some mothers do not lactate very well and anxiety in this case may interfere so much with the let-down reflex that the process becomes a vicious circle.

Once the baby goes onto formula and begins to be fully nourished, you can see her putting on weight and becoming more active and you will feel relieved that you have made the right decision. There is no reason why you cannot offer the breast to the baby if she will take it. There is never any need for a total break, although some mothers prefer it.

Persistent cracking of the nipples or persistent mastitis

Although these conditions can be dealt with, and ideally prevented, if they happen several times, you may find your powers of endurance giving out. You may have very sensitive nipples.

You may feel that for your own sake the baby should be on the bottle. Once the problem has passed, if you feel sad and regretful, try the baby at the breast. If this starts the trouble again, it is better to make the best of bottlefeeding. If you have another baby, read up on nipple and breast care in pregnancy (see pages 32–35), and try to identify what went wrong. Discuss it in advance with medical staff and breast-feeding experts, so that you are prepared.

Inability to cope with demand feeding

Although most babies will eventually find some pattern of feeding, some never do. Some mothers can cope with this, but some can't. You may feel you never know when the baby is going to wake for her next feed, and so you cannot organize your day. Your anxiety and inability to get organized may ruin your enjoyment of feeding and you may want to change to the bottle.

If you give up breastfeeding because of these apparently unending demands, you may rationalize this in a number of ways. Not having enough milk is one way – although your baby may be gaining weight and look bonny and happy. You may also be tempted to criticize breastfeeding generally. If the fact that you have failed to breastfeed makes you feel angry, bitter and resentful towards other mothers who seem to be coping with these demands, you need to work out exactly what you are so angry about and whether anything can be done to put it right. If not, it is best to put the anger out of your mind and enjoy bottlefeeding your baby.

Bad advice

Modern hospital practice can be instrumental in undermining your confidence and preventing the process of lactation from becoming established. You may be advised to give the baby complementary bottles, or you may be advised to abandon breastfeeding because of technical problems. Breastfeeding does not figure very largely in the training of doctors, and your doctor may not specialize in it. He may therefore give you inappropriate advice and you may give up breastfeeding unnecessarily.

If this has happened to you and you feel your advice was very bad and unsympathetic, you and your partner can write and complain. This will help to prevent other mothers from suffering the same experiences. Be polite and point out where the advice was wrong (if necessary quote a good medical text book – see page 126). You can get help on how to do this from one of the organizations listed on page 125.

If you have been advised to change to bottlefeeding, remember that you do not need to give up breastfeeding altogether. You can still put the baby to the breast. If you have given up and are very disappointed, you can even relactate with perseverance (see page 109).

Social pressures

You may have difficulty with in-laws living in the same house or a husband who is not enthusiastic about breastfeeding, or friends who send you upstairs to nurse when you visit. It is hard being the odd one out in a community that looks on bottlefeeding as the norm.

If you have succumbed to social pressures and regret it, try to think positively about feeding any future babies you may have. Get in touch with other people who look on breastfeeding as normal. You will then enjoy some moral support. Encourage your husband to think positively about breastfeeding too (see page 16).

Illness

A bout of flu or gastric infection may temporarily reduce the milk supply. Although breast milk is the best protection for your baby when there is infection around, you may feel that you just cannot manage feeding any more.

If your baby has become used to bottlefeeding, it may be kinder to continue with it rather than introduce too many changes of routine into her life. Some mothers feel relief when they turn to bottlefeeding. Some feel they have failed. (You can relactate when you feel better if you want to.)

If you feel like this, don't dwell on it; try instead to make bottlefeeding a success.

Successful bottlefeeding

The aims of successful bottlefeeding are the same as those for successful breastfeeding: a well-nourished, healthy infant and a happy feeding relationship between you and your baby – and in this case the father too. You do have to work just as hard. Be extra careful with sterilization (see page 83) and make conscious efforts to keep the baby near to you when you are feeding so that you both get the maximum enjoyment and mutual feedback from the experience. Hold the baby close to you just as you did when you were breastfeeding. You can even hold her next to your naked skin if you would like to.

Making bottlefeeding easier

Always make up the formula according to the manufacturer's instructions and never put in extra formula. This could lead to a concentration of minerals in the formula and hence the baby's bloodstream, which can lead to dehydration and illness. Choose the best formula for your baby and for your needs (take medical advice). You may choose one of the many powdered varieties, which include the so-called 'humanized' milks, scientifically modified so that they are as close to breast milk as possible; liquid formula, which is simple to measure and make up; or sealed, disposable bottles of ready-mixed formula. Whichever

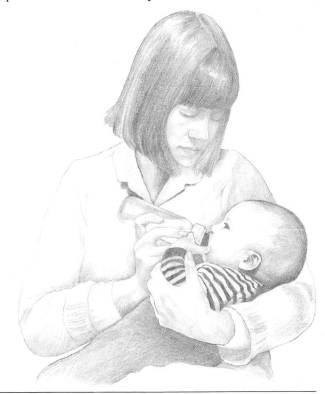

With the baby fairly upright in your arms, hold the bottle firmly and ensure that the teat is well back in her mouth. The teat should always be full of milk or the baby will take in too much air. If the teat flattens and no milk is getting through, pull the bottle gently back to release the vacuum.

formula you choose that is best for your baby, keep to the same proprietary brand.

When you are preparing the formula, make up a bit more than your baby is likely to need – but if she doesn't finish it, throw it away. A bottlefed baby can also be irregular in her feeding demands. Some mothers make up a large jug of formula and keep it covered in the refrigerator, transferring it to sterile bottles at feed times as needed. Therefore, if the baby wants eight smallish feeds rather than five large ones, she can have them on demand.

Have a least eight to ten bottles in the sterilizer so that you don't have to re-sterilize them during the day. It can then all be done at the end of the day.

When you are feeding the baby, hold the bottle at an angle so that the teat is well back in her mouth and it always has milk in it; this way the baby will swallow less air and have less wind. (If the teat is not flowing fast enough – several drops per second – enlarge the hole with a red-hot needle.) Let the baby have breaks from the feeding now and then. Don't add extra cereal to her bottle in the hope that she will sleep longer. It will just make her fat. If she is hungry, offer her more milk. She will not need solids until she is four to six months old. Bottlefed babies may sometimes need drinks of water though, especially in hot weather.

Enjoy your baby in all the other ways you can. Feeding is an important part of life in the early weeks – but as the baby grows and develops, it becomes progressively less important. Smiles, sounds, play and the increasing control your baby shows over her environment will all provide new opportunities for you to build up your relationship. There is never any need for a mother who is enjoying and encouraging all these aspects of her baby's development to feel a failure. A healthy responsive baby is a success, however she is fed.

Sterilizing

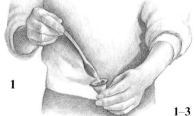

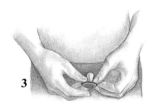

1–3 To clean the teat, pour a little salt into it. Roll the teat between your fingers to clear any slime, then rinse under running cold water. Turn the teat inside out to check for any salt and mucus.

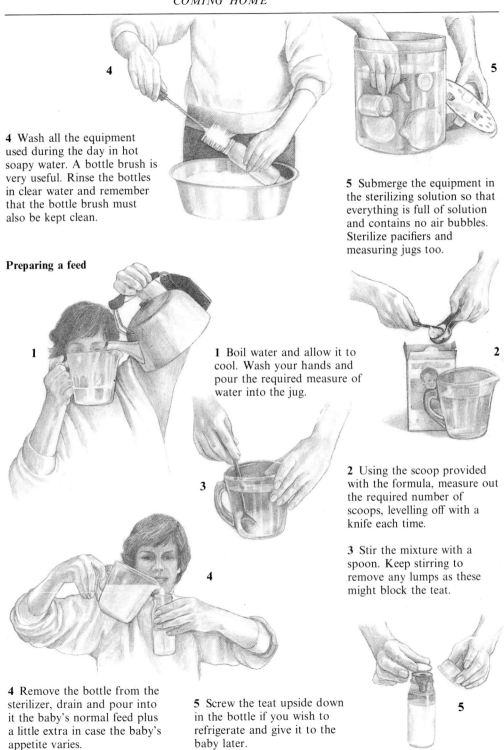

4 Wash all the equipment used during the day in hot soapy water. A bottle brush is very useful. Rinse the bottles in clear water and remember that the bottle brush must also be kept clean.

5 Submerge the equipment in the sterilizing solution so that everything is full of solution and contains no air bubbles. Sterilize pacifiers and measuring jugs too.

Preparing a feed

1 Boil water and allow it to cool. Wash your hands and pour the required measure of water into the jug.

2 Using the scoop provided with the formula, measure out the required number of scoops, levelling off with a knife each time.

3 Stir the mixture with a spoon. Keep stirring to remove any lumps as these might block the teat.

4 Remove the bottle from the sterilizer, drain and pour into it the baby's normal feed plus a little extra in case the baby's appetite varies.

5 Screw the teat upside down in the bottle if you wish to refrigerate and give it to the baby later.

6 *THE BREASTFEEDING FAMILY*

The focus up to now has been on the mother and the baby. The first part of this chapter is addressed to the father, a very important person in the breastfeeding family.

Adjustment to fatherhood

If you have involved yourself with your wife's pregnancy and been with her for the delivery, this is a good preparation for being a 'breastfeeding father'. However, antenatal care, antenatal classes and the process of childbirth – even where fathers are involved – all tend to reinforce the importance of the mother and baby. Being required to give support all the time can put a strain on you, the father. Other fathers may help; but don't forget your partner. Although she is pre-occupied with her own and the baby's condition, you are still the most important adult person in her life. If you feel insufficiently informed, or left out, confide in her.

Breastfeeding extends this central role of motherhood beyond birth. Only the woman can breastfeed. Does this matter to the father? Unfortunately, there is little proper evidence about fathers' attitudes and behaviour when it comes to breastfeeding. It is often said that fathers are possessive about their wives' breasts and may be jealous of the baby; it is also said that fathers who can bottlefeed must be closer to their babies – but there is a lack of convincing evidence to back these theories up. What research there is shows that fathers are very important people to the breast-feeding mother. In one major study, the father's attitude was the most important source of influence, after the mother's own views, in deciding whether to breastfeed. The same study found that fathers were also the biggest source of help after the birth; 81 per cent of mothers had help from fathers, with relatives and friends quite a long way behind.

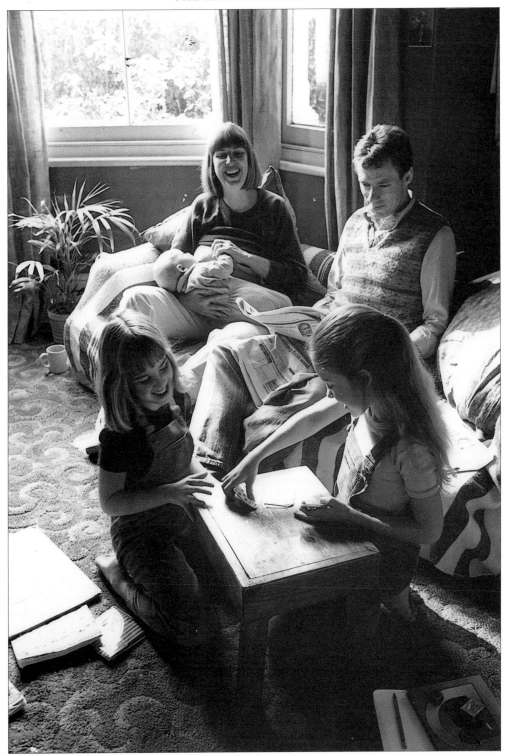

Problems in perspective	If you find it a problem having a nursing mother around the house, instead of the independent person your wife was before, it can help to remember two things: first, bottlefeeding fathers have to face similar changes in their wives; and second, there are two ways of looking at a problem. It might turn out to be an advantage, looked at in a different light.

Problem	A different perspective
Your wife's body is still claimed by the baby. Her breasts seem exclusively for him; they look different, they may be sore, or leaking. She seems distant and less attractive. She may still be overweight after the birth and this is depressing for her.	Her body is functioning perfectly if she is successfully nursing your baby. This is something to be proud of. Breast changes and discomfort can be distressing for the mother. Be sympathetic and remind her that it will pass. Many men love to watch their women nursing their babies. One doctor who has worked extensively with psychosexual problems claims that men do not notice changes in the bodies of the women they love as much as the women think they do. Many of the changes are attractive. Even if they are not, reassure your wife that she is lovely and lovable.
Your wife is totally involved with caring for your baby. You feel less important and you can't do any of the feeding.	Some people might say that this is an advantage because it lets fathers off the hook. This is a limited view. Your baby is getting the best possible nourishment which will protect his health both now and in the future. Remember that babies enjoy other things – being held, rocked, sung and talked to. When the mother is tired and tense, you have the advantage of not being so intensely involved. You can help to calm both her and the baby.
Your wife's emotional state fluctuates. She may be positive and then drained of confidence. She is susceptible to critical remarks made by other people, including you, and she loses her temper easily. She is still tired after the birth, and feeding problems or her stitches may be troubling her.	Living with a new mother in this frame of mind can be like living with several different people. Try to look at this positively; enjoy her cheerful moods, and stay calm during her depression. She needs to be reassured that life can still be normal; your staying as normal as possible will help. Protect her from the criticism of others. Enjoy being needed and important to her. This includes practical tasks around the house.
The housework is never done; the meals are never properly prepared or cooked. You have no ironed shirts. Your wife is doing	Try to see the light side. It really doesn't matter if the house is untidy for a few weeks. If it is getting you down, perhaps you could pay someone to help out for a period. If not, use laundries, convenience foods and disposables of every description. Concentrate on priorities; you may find this a

nothing for you because she's feeding every two hours, and when she isn't feeding she is resting, eating, drinking or bathing. You are expected to go to work and carry on as normal.

Dos and don'ts

valuable exercise in deciding just what is important. Enjoying your baby and your new status as a family can bring new and different pleasures.

If you should feel resentful, tell your wife. You can discuss your feelings and work out your priorities much better together. Try to get a good night's sleep, perhaps sleep in another room; there is no point in both of you being tired.

Praise your wife and say she's doing well, even if you don't think so. If you have sought information on breastfeeding and baby behaviour, when she gets things out of perspective, you will be better able to remind her of the facts. It would help if you took some regular responsibility for the baby, such as taking him out for a walk.

In these early days the domestic routine probably won't run smoothly. See to your own clothes and those of any other children. Don't keep asking 'Are you sure he's getting enough?' or let others do so, and never say 'My mother/sister/girlfriend/ex-wife managed to breastfeed, so why can't you?'

Tenderness and rapport can develop from birth between a father and his baby when they have regular contact with each other.

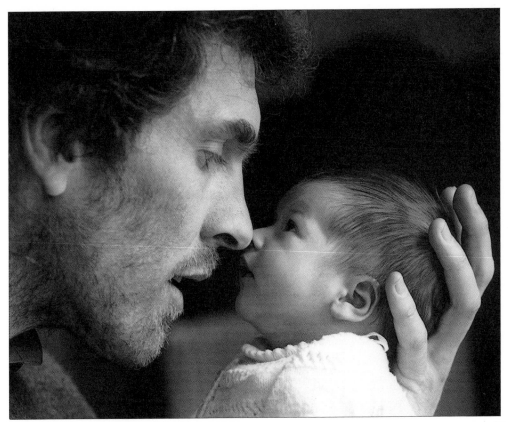

Older children

Much of the writing about introducing a new baby to an older child or children concentrates on jealousy. It is obvious that the arrival of a new baby has a big impact on a small child's life in all sorts of ways. Mother is tired and cumbersome during pregnancy; she disappears into hospital to have the baby; strange people visit the house; dad is doing the cooking; somebody else's mother is picking him up from playgroup. If an adult's life were suddenly disrupted in all these ways, we wouldn't be a bit surprised if the adult objected. Be understanding of any resentment, but don't let him get away with too much or he really will feel that something is wrong.

Nevertheless, many young children react extremely well to the arrival of a new baby, so long as the period while the mother is away is managed well, with a familiar person caring for the child and plenty of preparation about babies in general and the new baby in particular. Babies can be fascinating to children. There is no doubt that, once the baby learns to look around and distinguish particular familiar faces, the older child's is one that he will especially delight in. Many first smiles are bestowed on big brother or sister. The jealousy problem, if it is there and so long as the parents do not draw too much attention to it, may be solved by the baby.

Does this make breastfeeding more difficult?

Some surveys show that mothers who have had babies before are less likely than first-time mothers to start breastfeeding. This probably reflects the number of women

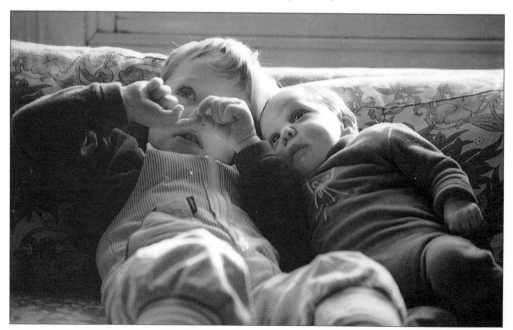

who found breastfeeding difficult and were happier to change to bottlefeeding. Some mothers who failed to breastfeed for long previously are eager to succeed next time. A few mothers, who were successful breastfeeders with their first babies, worry that they won't manage it so well with the second and fear that breastfeeding will upset the older child more than bottlefeeding would. Should they bottlefeed instead? If you are such a mother, you may gain reassurance from some research that studied the impact of a second baby on 40 families. Roughly half the families were breastfeeding and half bottlefeeding. The researchers found that the older children were more likely to try to irritate the bottlefed babies than the breastfed ones.

Many mothers find that lactation goes more smoothly with second and later children; they seem to have more milk and suffer from fewer technical problems. If you had sore nipples or mastitis last time, you will know how to identify the problem early and prevent it.

Whatever your feelings and worries about your older child or children, it would be unfair to deny your second child the advantages of breastfeeding (see pages 8–11). A subsequent child misses out on the attention the first child had. But, if he is breastfed, he will at least be cuddled and held close to you a few times a day. Nursing him and watching his responses will give you valuable information about his personality.

If you failed to breastfeed your first child, and are now successfully feeding your second, you may feel guilty that you are giving the second baby something you didn't give to the first. There is no need to. First children get all that undivided attention from their parents that subsequent children obviously cannot get, however much they are loved.

Tandem nursing

This term is used when a woman continues to breastfeed an older child after a second (or subsequent) child is born. Should you continue breastfeeding the older one if you become pregnant while nursing? The answer can depend on the age of the child. If he is still only a few months old, he will be relying on breast milk for some, if not all, of his nourishment. Pregnancy can cause a diminution of the milk supply because of the extra hormones, especially oestrogen, that are circulating in the mother's body. This may mean that you *have* to introduce your older one to other foods but there is no reason why you should not go on suckling him for comfort if you both want to.

If the child is older – say nine to twelve months or more – breastfeeding will be more for comfort than nutrition. It is not strictly necessary for the child's physical well-being, but

From an early age big brother or sister can be a conspirator and friend – and a comfortable cushion.

if you both enjoy it, there is no need to stop. If you feel that you would rather wean the older one so that you can concentrate your physical and mental energies on the coming baby, then try to do so gently.

Towards the end of pregnancy, your milk supply may increase again and your breasts will be making colostrum. Colostrum and transitional milk are different from mature milk (see pages 26–27) – and the new baby should get this milk because he needs it most. If you are still nursing your older child after the baby is born, make sure that the baby is adequately fed first and let your older one have his comfort suck afterwards. Some children want more nursing at this time; some wean themselves and become more grown-up.

You need to see to your own needs above all. Make sure you are well nourished – vitamin supplements, therefore, are recommended. If you are happy with what you are doing, ignore ill-informed criticism. If you are not happy and would like to stop feeding the older one, don't feel guilty about doing so. The children's well-being depends on yours and the older child won't like being resented. Find other ways of giving him attention.

Occasionally an older child who has been weaned will want to copy the new baby and have a suck at the breast. You can let him if you want – but remember that children quickly forget how to 'milk' the breast with the proper sucking technique. If you don't want to, say 'breastfeeding is not for big boys' and offer him some other treat instead.

How to cope with other children
Fixed points in the day

Some things are always done at a regular time, such as taking a child to school or playgroup, or sitting down to watch television, so plan round them. Feed the baby half an hour before you have to go out, even if he's not demanding it; it's better than having him screaming while you are delayed by the teacher or other parents. Feed the baby before the older child's special time or bedtime so that you know you can give the older child some attention. Demand feeding, after the first two weeks or so, usually has to be modified with second or later babies. Feeding in advance is usually better than trying to make the baby wait.

Offers of help

Accept all the help that is offered and don't be shy about asking for it. But try not to let other people take the older child away too much. He will know that he's seen as a nuisance and will understandably resent it. A planned visit or outing with a good friend is different. Try to arrange for such visits before the baby arrives, then use this time to get acquainted with the baby and to have a rest.

Help from older children

Enlist the older child's help as much as you can, giving him praise and the occasional reward for being sensible and grown-up. Some children behave more babyishly for a while after a new baby arrives; but many actually progress faster and start doing things for themselves. Encourage this – even if he isn't very efficient. A toddler can fetch a tissue, alert you to the doorbell, tell you if the baby is crying or pick up a rattle from the floor. Older childen, particularly school-age ones, can help with household chores, cuddle and rock the baby and do things for themselves. All this is to be encouraged; it will make them better able to look after themselves and to be more competent parents in their turn.

Older children can learn about parenthood naturally if they share in the closeness of nursing with the mother and baby.

Breastfeeding a baby in front of older children is the easiest and most natural way for young people to learn about breastfeeding – and the children usually take it completely for granted. So do their friends from bottlefeeding families, once the novelty has worn off.

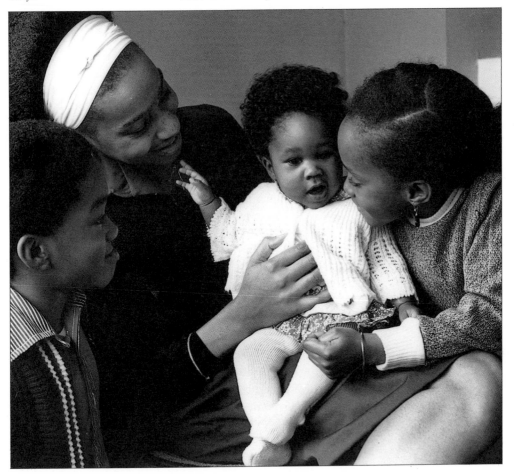

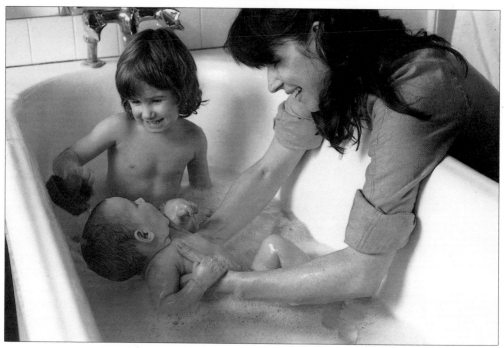

You can save time, energy and hot water by bathing the children together – and they have fun too.

Second babies are often very 'good' and undemanding; they have to be, as research shows that their mothers are much less responsive to them than they are to first babies. However, if you have one that refuses to be overlooked in this way, put him in a baby chair or bouncing cradle within sight of the older children so that they can cheer him up. Carrying him around in a sling can also be effective.

Being part of the family

Do as much as you can for the children together. It's probably better if feeding and meals don't coincide at first – but when the baby starts on solids, he should join the family. Baby and older child can be bathed together and they don't have to be bathed every day. Try to get naps, bedtimes and outings to coincide as much as possible. Boost your supply, if you need to, by nursing while you sit and watch television with the older child or while reading a story. But do try to set aside one time each day when the older child has your undivided attention: a bedtime story, or an afternoon snack.

Rest

Try to catch up on some sleep. The study about the impact of second babies (see page 89) found that most mothers got only five and a half hours sleep in 24 hours – and this was broken. If you can, go back to bed after breakfast while the older child is at playgroup. If your older child is under playgroup age, rest when he lies down for his afternoon nap. You can always do the housework while he's up and about.

Otherwise, try to get to bed earlier in the evening, again waking the baby and feeding him first. Do everything you can sitting down. Don't take on other responsibilities for the first few weeks after the birth.

Other members of the family
Older women

Your mother and mother-in-law probably fed their children in a different manner from the way in which you will be feeding your baby. If they bottlefed, or breastfed according to a rigid schedule, they may feel threatened by your approach to breastfeeding. It may seem an implied criticism of them and they may unwittingly make comments that seem to undermine you, for example: 'Wasn't he fed only two hours ago?' or, more subtly, 'You poor girl, you're wearing yourself out'.

If older members of the family say things like this, try not to be resentful about it. Try to understand the different circumstances in which they brought up their babies. Despite differences in child-rearing and feeding styles, some aspects of babycare always stay the same. Ask for the advice and support of the older generation in every way you can – if necessary, steering clear of feeding. Grandmothers can give a lot of help in practical ways. Asking for the benefits of their experience can bring you closer in ways that will be valuable to you all. Many mothers who have been rather distant from their own parents find that a baby brings them closer.

Even if you don't get on with the older generation, remember that your children won't feel the same way. Children deserve the love and company of their grand-parents and other family members. The extended family may be more scattered nowadays but its value and usefulness can be as great as ever if you keep up the contacts. Same-generation contacts can provide a valuable breastfeeding support group; if your sisters or cousins breastfed their babies, you have a better chance of breastfeeding yours.

Older men in the family

A reason sometimes given for not breastfeeding is the mother's embarrassment at the thought of feeding in front of her father-in-law (or, indeed, in front of her own father), where she and her husband are living with in-laws. This is an understandable feeling, but it need not be as big a problem as you think. In the first place, many older men are more familiar with the sight of a baby being breastfed than younger men are. It may not bother them at all. If *you* are bothered, you can easily arrange to feed the baby in another room when grandfather is around. If you are living with the older generation, presumably you will have your own room; arrange things so that you can feed the baby there.

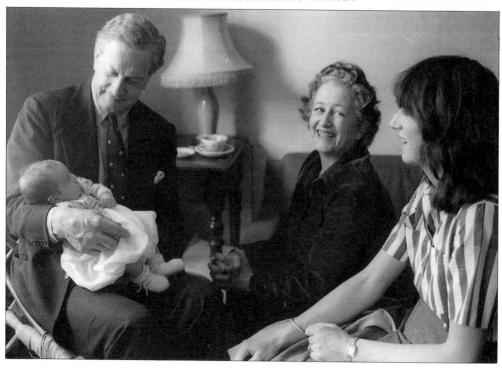

Grandparents provide interesting new faces and voices which help to enlarge the baby's social world.

Many parents are proud of their daughter's ability to breastfeed and will do a great deal to support you and praise you. If you know you are going to have a lot of contact with your parents and parents-in-law after the baby comes, it is important to discuss feeding with them during pregnancy.

Sexuality and breastfeeding

Lactation and breastfeeding are part of women's sexual functioning and this association is probably the reason why some people see breastfeeding as lovely and sensuous while others think it distasteful. Lactation is controlled by the hormones that influence other sexual activities – particularly the hormone oxytocin, which initiates the let-down reflex and is released during both labour and orgasm. The breasts are an erogenous zone that is attractive to both men and women. They are very sensitive to contact, particularly the nipple area (see page 20); some women enjoy this contact and can achieve orgasm from it. Others positively dislike it and prefer other parts of their bodies to be caressed and stimulated. Not liking to have your breasts touched does not mean that you are sexually frigid; nor does it mean that you can't breastfeed. The sexual aspect of breastfeeding does produce ambivalent feelings, however, and reactions to it manifest themselves in many ways.

Embarrassment and
revulsion

The fact that so many women choose to bottlefeed because they would find breastfeeding embarrassing has to be taken seriously, but it is not necessarily a problem in practice. In one survey of women who doubted the arguments for breastfeeding but nevertheless tried it, the women found breastfeeding less embarrassing and inconvenient than they had expected. Other research shows that reasons for giving up (see pages 78–80) are usually technical (insufficient milk, sore nipples and so on), and not because of embarrassment.

Although breastfeeding is sexual and can provide physical feelings of great sensuality and enjoyment to the mother and, no doubt, to the baby, its sexual nature needs to be kept in perspective. There are women who report achieving orgasm during breastfeeding. But, if you breastfeed for, say, nine months, you are going to be giving your baby around 1500 breastfeeds. You cannot maintain a level of orgasmic ecstasy when you are doing something as often and routinely as that.

Breastfeeding is sometimes compared to lovemaking. It is a close intimate physical relationship, but it is primarily a way of giving milk and immunological protection to a young baby, and, as is Nature's way, pleasure is thrown in as a bonus to ensure that this life-sustaining process continues. Unlike the mutual give-and-take of a successful adult relationship, breastfeeding often has to take place at inconvenient times and at the inconvenience of one or other of the participants. The baby may demand feeding when the mother does not find it convenient to comply. If the mother's breasts are overfull, she may get the baby to meet her needs by helping to empty them. The activity of breastfeeding, unlike lovemaking, often takes place in unromantic and non-intimate circumstances.

Breastfeeding is often promoted in a romanticized way in photographs showing mother and baby naked with the emphasis placed on the sensuality (but also surely on the inconvenience – imagine breastfeeding your baby with no nappy on every time). It is understandable that, seeing such promotions, some women fear that it will be both embarrassing and inconvenient. Breastfeeding can bring real pleasure – but the normal part it plays in everyday life needs to be stressed too, particularly to the large number of people who are embarrassed about it.

Feelings while you feed

The physical processes that make breastfeeding pleasurable for mother and baby (see pages 10–11) will not be the same at every feed. However, the circulation of prolactin in your body may have a generally calming effect on you. When oxytocin is released to get the let-down reflex going, you may feel a tension in your breasts as the milk starts to flow, and then a pleasant feeling of relaxation as the tension subsides and the baby nurses. These feelings can come quite unexpectedly; you may have been tearing around and feel quite resentful that the baby has woken up just 20 minutes too early. Nursing can help you relax. Once breastfeeding is well established, the inhibitory effect of tension on the let-down seems to be less likely. Many mothers report that often, when they are breastfeeding in situations of great stress, exhaustion, hurry and furtiveness, the process almost seems to work in reverse, with the let-down *producing* feelings of relaxation.

Intimate moments

There will be times, of course, when breastfeeding your baby has a special, intimate, loving quality – when you seem to be as close as you can possibly be to anyone. Perhaps it will be at night, when your baby snuggles up close to you and nurses blissfully while your partner puts his arms around you both. Perhaps it will be when the baby is a few weeks old and suddenly comes off the breast, looks straight at you and gives you that first, real, eye-to-eye smile, then carries on nursing again. It may be when he is a few months old and reaches up with his hands to pat and stroke you. Such moments are all the more precious for not being commonplace.

Women vary enormously in their emotional and physical reactions to their experiences. Babies vary a lot, too. You may feel the most sensuous woman in the world yet have a businesslike baby who wolfs his feed down in three minutes flat on one side and two minutes on the other and then has had enough. It is no use hoping for a languorous nursing session if the baby won't co-operate. On the other hand, you may see breastfeeding only as a practical way of giving your baby the best nourishment.

If you're somebody who fears the intimacy and physicality of breastfeeding and the embarrassment of doing it – remember that these fears don't seem to matter very much to other women once they've had a baby. If you're a woman who gets enormous sensuous pleasure out of nursing and for whom breastfeeding is going well, with a lot of support and admiration from your husband or partner, then you are fortunate indeed. Whatever your feelings, try not to be critical of other women who don't feel about breastfeeding the way you do.

Other people's attitudes

When breastfeeding is seen as a pleasant, convenient and healthy way of feeding a baby, there can be no possible objection to a mother breastfeeding her baby as long as they both want. No-one thinks it odd that toddlers suck on thumbs or pacifiers until they are two, three or older, so why should there be anything odd about breastfeeding then?

Unfortunately, some people do not see it this way, and these may include your doctor and other medical advisers. They see the advantages of breast *milk* for the newborn baby – but breast*feeding* an older baby can seem to them an indecent act. Many mothers are pressured to wean their babies after four to six months for this reason.

Such attitudes reveal much about the sexual anxieties of the people who hold them. Oddly though, there do not seem to be the same objections to the fact that mothers change their babies and thus have to handle their babies' genitals as many times a day as they breastfeed – sometimes more often. Nobody suggests that this kind of intimate handling – and the kissing, caressing and holding that are a normal part of childcare – should not continue after four to six months. There is absolutely no sexual reason why breastfeeding should not continue after this either. In most parts of the world – and until this century, in all parts of the world – children have been breastfed until two, three, four years of age as a matter of course.

Sex with your partner

Some surveys have suggested that breastfeeding mothers are more eager to resume sexual intercourse after the birth than are bottlefeeders. This may be because of the sexual hormonal activity; it may, of course, be because these women are more physical in the first place, with greater enjoyment of their bodily functions, which is why they both chose to breastfeed and to resume intercourse.

Possible problems

Some newly delivered women can be at a disadvantage when it comes to resuming intercourse. Many will have had episiotomies during the birth and will still be suffering tenderness, if not pain, where they were stitched. For some unfortunate women this pain can go on for weeks, or even months. Another side-effect can be dryness in the vagina; the normal lubricants are not produced so efficiently.

The breasts too may be tender, particularly in the first few weeks. When they are full of milk, they may feel hard and lumpy and any pressure on them causes pain. Milk can also leak out of them, either as a result of pressure when they are full of milk or during orgasm when the release of oxytocin produces a let-down reflex. For all these reasons, both you and your partner may be nervous about touching them. They are also rather inaccessible if you are wearing a nursing bra at night to hold the breast pads in place if you leak or if your breasts are feeling heavy and uncomfortable.

A quiet cuddle at night can soothe the baby so he is calm for his feed.

As well as all this, you will still be getting back to normal after the efforts of childbirth and your stay in hospital, and neither of you will probably be getting much sleep. Also the baby demands a great deal of attention and affection. It all adds up to a situation that may not be ideal for lovemaking.

Resuming lovemaking

You may be advised not to have intercourse until after your six-week, post-delivery check-up. However, if your vagina and perineum feel comfortable and both of you want to make love, there is no reason why you shouldn't do so. If your stitches still feel tender and your breasts are uncomfortable, there is no need to abandon all displays of affection and desire. Other parts of yours and your partner's body can be caressed and kissed; you are both in need of tender, loving care at this time. You can express this with each other, even without full intercourse.

Lubrication of the vagina with a contraceptive gel can make you more comfortable and if your partner is gentle and patient, intercourse may still be successful even while your perineum is not completely normal. You may need to experiment with positions; anything too strenuous for you or that puts pressure on your breasts needs to be avoided to start with.

To prevent leaking, which may occur at orgasm and can be off-putting (although some couples find it quite exciting), try to feed the baby before you make love, even if he doesn't particularly want to be fed. Babies and small children seem to have an uncanny instinct for waking up at the most sensitive moments. If having the baby in the room is distracting, put his crib elsewhere temporarily.

If you do leak, it's a wise precaution to have a towel on the bed to protect the sheets. All these anxieties about leaking and mess and extra protections may seem off-putting to you; but like any aspect of your life together, however unromantic, they can be included in your expressions of affection for each other. Leaking breasts and towels may not be the height of eroticism but you can laugh together about them and recognize, again, that they are a sign that your body is functioning beautifully, as a healthy female body should after a baby has just been born.

Contraception

If you are breastfeeding your baby on demand, with no complementary bottles or other foods, the high levels of prolactin in your body help to suppress ovulation. On average, it can take six to eight months for periods to return in women who breastfeed unrestrictedly for the first few months. In women who don't breastfeed, or who practise

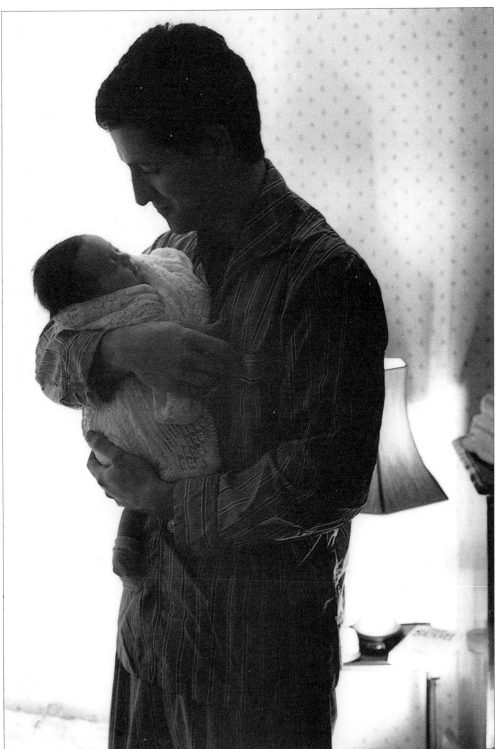

token, infrequent, supplemented breastfeeding, the average time for the return of their periods is two to four months. These are averages of course; you may find that, even when you have introduced solid foods and drinks from cups, but are still nursing, your periods don't come back for a year or more. On the other hand, you may be fully breastfeeding and your periods will return after only a few weeks.

In some new mothers, ovulation occurs before menstruation. So you can be producing eggs and therefore be capable of conceiving, even before you have had a period. Some mothers do this and go from one baby to another, with as much as a two-year gap between babies, without ever having a period at all. In some women, the first period or two may be 'anovular', that is, no eggs have been produced, but the body still menstruates.

Can breastfeeding stop you conceiving?

Statistically the long period of time when lactating women are not ovulating helps to prevent more pregnancies than all other types of contraceptive device put together – on a worldwide scale. But statistics tell us only about large groups; individuals vary and you therefore cannot rely on breastfeeding to act as a contraceptive for *you*.

If you have religious objections to artificial contraception, full, natural breastfeeding may help to delay your next pregnancy. The drawback is that you cannot use the rhythm method, or 'safe period', since, while you are not ovulating or having any periods, you cannot measure your temperature and ovulation patterns.

The pill

Contraceptive pills containing oestrogen may reduce milk production. The amount of oestrogen in the pill has been progressively reduced over the past few years as it has been found to have other undesirable side-effects. If you are breastfeeding and want to take the pill, you will probably be prescribed a progestogen-only pill (the mini-pill), which does not reduce the milk supply – it may even boost it. On the other hand, it is not quite as reliable a contraceptive as the combined, low-oestrogen/progestogen pill. Nevertheless, combined with the reduced fertility produced by breastfeeding, the progestogen-only pill has been a satisfactory contraceptive for many breastfeeding women. When you visit the family planning clinic, be sure to tell the doctor that you are breastfeeding and ask for his or her advice.

The pill will either be prescribed before you leave hospital or at your six-week, post-partum check-up. If you want to have intercourse before the check-up, it would b᷉ ᷉e to use another contraceptive method. One drawba͟c͟k ᷉ ᷉e pill is that its hormones are secreted in the milk and it is not certain what effect this has on the baby. No ill-effects have been reported so far, but studies are still in their early stages. If you go back on the pill, and then find that your baby is more fretful and not gaining so much weight as before, consider coming off the pill and trying another contraceptive method if you want to keep your supply.

Contraceptive injections

There has been much controversy in the past few years about the use of injectable steroids (under the name Depo-Provera) for long-term contraception in newly delivered mothers. The effect of these injections can last up to three months, or up to six months. They *may* reduce the quantity and/or quality of the milk; the evidence is not conclusive one way or the other. We also do not know what effect such powerful drugs may have on the baby. If other methods of contraception are acceptable, they are preferable. Depo-Provera is sometimes given routinely to new mothers in conjunction with the rubella vaccine – and these women may not even be told that they have been given this drug. This practice is completely indefensible. If you are advised to have rubella vaccine (and, of course, it is important you don't conceive while the vaccine is still active because rubella harms unborn babies), make sure that you are given no other injection without your knowledge.

Other contraceptive methods

The intrauterine device (IUD) can be fitted at or after your six-week check-up, provided that all is well and any stitches or infections you may have are healed. The IUD may even help to boost your milk supply by stimulating the womb and encouraging the production of oxytocin. However, if you have not used one before, you might prefer to wait until you have finished breastfeeding before having one fitted, using another method meanwhile.

Barrier methods, although less sophisticated and requiring more effort, may suit the needs of the breastfeeding family best during the early months. They have no side-effects; they can be used 'on demand', which may be more suitable for the somewhat erratic nature of the sexual behaviour of new parents. Contraceptive gels and creams can also be used for lubricating the vagina. If you use a cap, or diaphragm, your pre-pregnancy one won't do. You may need to be measured more than once for a new one as you regain your non-pregnant state inside.

An advantage of the sheath, or condom, is that the man is taking some of the responsibility at a time when responsibilities of all kinds are very heavy on the nursing mother. Whatever method you use, you should, of course, be in agreement about it.

7 *THE GROWING BABY*

In the first three months babies gain, on average, about 200 g (7 oz) per week. In the second three months, they slow down and put on an average 110–140 g (4–5 oz) per week. In the second half of the first year, their growth rate slows down even more – an average of 100 g ($3\frac{1}{2}$ oz) per week. Thus, while the baby is being fed primarily on milk (whether breast or bottle), her rate of growth is actually faster than it is when she starts having a wider variety of other solid and semi-solid foods in the second six months.

The rate of growth is not the same for every baby. It also depends on her size at birth and what size she is genetically destined to be. If she was very tiny at birth, say, below 2.2 kg (5 lb), she will double her birthweight sooner than a 4.5 kg (10 lb) birthweight baby, who may not reach the weight of 9 kg (20 lb) until she is nearly a year old.

Feeding patterns

There comes a point in the first three months when your baby becomes a settled individual. You have ceased to worry about what time she will wake up and whether your milk supply is going to disappear. At this stage, you and your baby will have developed your own feeding routine. Breast-feeding is a dyadic form of behaviour, in which both partners interact and respond closely with one another. Babies do fit in with the kinds of mothers they have, and mothers do the same for their babies. There is no right pattern – the pattern you and your baby arrive at is right for you.

Sometimes it can take longer to synchronize your behaviour. This can happen even with breastfeeding mothers who are supposedly in tune with their babies' needs, especially if you have a wakeful, demanding baby. If you feel that you and your baby are not getting on as well as you would like, then do seek help and don't struggle on alone.

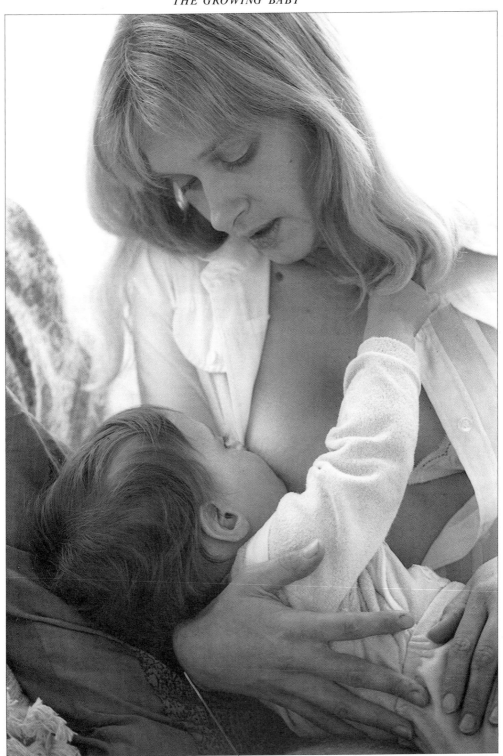

Problems with the growing baby

Problem	Symptoms	Causes
Growth spurt	This often occurs at around 12 weeks. A settled baby suddenly becomes more demanding; wants more frequent feeding and more night feeds.	Babies don't grow and develop at the same rate. A slow growth period may be followed by a spurt in demand. She may be using up more energy.
Fluctuation in milk supply or a noticeable drop	The baby is more demanding but has slow or no weight gain. Drier nappies, infrequent, scanty bowel movements. You can feel that you don't have much milk. The let-down is less noticeable.	A growth spurt in the baby may coincide with more demands being made on you. You may not be eating enough. You may be rushing around and have let the baby go too long between feeds so that she's only having 3 or 4 per day.
		You have gone back on the pill.
		Introduction of solids too quickly.
Reluctance to feed	The baby spends only 2 or 3 minutes at each breast, then wriggles and cries to get down. Doesn't want to comfort suck any more.	The baby is by now an efficient feeder and gets all the milk she needs in this time.
Nursing strike	The baby refuses the breast altogether. May scream and protest or not be interested.	Mysterious. The baby may be responding to stress in you, or menstruation or even an unfamiliar perfume. She may not be hungry.
	The baby may be listless, have unusual bowel movements, or a runny nose.	The baby may be ill.
Night waking	The baby wakes at some time in the night, wanting attention and feeding.	Some babies take many months to sleep through the night. She may be hungry because she is not being fed often enough during the day. She may just want comfort. She may not have learned the difference between day and night.
	The baby starts to wake in the night after having slept through for a while.	She may be hungry.
		The baby is teething or in pain. She may be distressed after some new experience in the day.
Teething and biting	Teeth appear; the baby's gums may be sore, she may dribble a lot, and want to gnaw things. She may be fretful and have red patches on her cheeks.	Natural development which varies from baby to baby. Some get their first teeth at 3 months, others not until a year or more. Many symptoms are blamed on teething.
	The baby may bite the breast.	Playfulness in the baby. Biting is a natural by-product of teeth but it is not an efficient way of getting milk from the breast.

Solutions

Boost your supply by giving the extra feeds that the baby demands. These demands will subside in a few days. Check the weight gain. You may find that after this period it has gone up. If the baby is over 4 months, this may be a cue for solid foods.

Increase your calorie intake, take things easy for a day or two. Give some extra feeds to boost your supply. If you find you have no milk at all at any time, you will need to give something else. Use stored breast milk or an approved formula. Don't worry; the milk will usually return. If it does not, you may have to wean the baby onto other milk foods, but you can still suckle her.

Reconsider your contraceptive method (see page 101).

Always offer the breast first, give 1 or 2 extra feeds and fewer solids. Solids are better introduced gradually (see page 122).

If her weight gain, nappies and behaviour are all normal, your baby has had enough to eat. There may still be times when she wants to nurse longer again (when she is tired or frightened).

Check whether your behaviour has become more tense. Try to put this right. Feed the baby when she is calm or has just woken up. Express to get your let-down going, and then feed her. Change feeding positions. Don't panic.

See your doctor. You may need to give extra fluids in a bottle or by spoon if she continues to refuse the breast. Express or pump your milk and freeze or refrigerate it to give to her.

If you want to persuade your baby to sleep at night, try to make night feeds as quiet and brief as possible. Don't turn on the light or change her. Leaving her to cry is distressing. Some babies may respond to being ignored; you know your baby best. Make sure she has a good feed before you go to bed. Try changing her sleeping arrangements. Put her in a larger crib. Cut down on her sleep during the day.

If this happens between 3 to 5 months, it could be a growth spurt. This requires extra feeding or the introduction of solids.

Nursing is the best comfort for a baby in pain or distress.

Some babies are soothed by extra nursing when their gums are sore. Something cool on the gums may help (ice packs or a chilled water-filled teething rattle). Teething gels may work. If the baby is in obvious pain, see your doctor. Give her plenty of hard, smooth objects to gnaw and bite on.

This is very painful. Remove her from the breast and say 'no' firmly. Watch her as you feed and remove the nipple as soon as it is obvious the milk is no longer flowing. It is not necessary to wean when the baby gets teeth. It could be a cue for solids though.

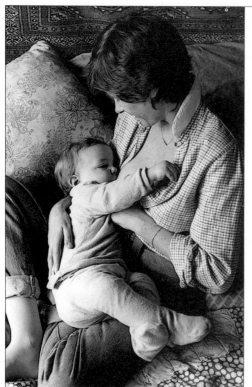

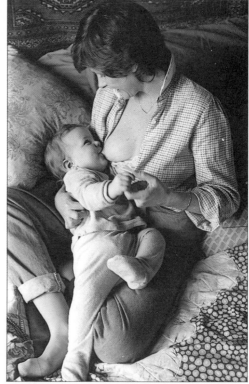

The nursing one-year-old and his mother are now perfectly attuned to each other. Nursing provides a comforting drink and an opportunity for play. When his thirst and need for a suck are satisfied, the baby then decides that it is time for a chat and a chuckle. His mother picks up his cue; if he wants to laugh, then he is in a good position for tickling. And the breast is still there if he becomes tired of playing and wants a comforting drink again.

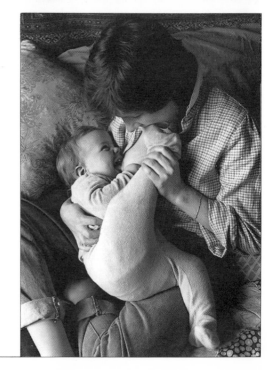

Advantages of feeding the older baby

As the baby grows, she shows more signs both of her individual personality and her developing maturity. She becomes more patient and more easily distracted; she can wait for her feed if there is an interesting toy, or person, or game to be enjoyed.

Play and convenience

Even in the very early days, the alternating sucking and pausing pattern of feeding is like a dialogue. The older baby develops this into real conversation and play during breast-feeding. Not every feed will be a leisurely playtime. Some are short and allow you to do other things at the same time. If your baby has hurt herself or she finds the irritation of teething unpleasant, the breast is always there as a source of reassurance.

Going into hospital

Your baby

If your baby has to go into hospital, you should make every effort to be admitted with her. This is true for all mothers but particularly for breastfeeding mothers. When a baby is ill, she most needs the comfort of a familiar and loved face. A baby who is friendly with strangers at other times won't be when she is in distress. Emotionally and physically she will be less disturbed if she is not missing you.

If you are breastfeeding, the breast milk provides extra protection against infection (and there are many infections in hospitals) and nursing gives comfort too. You will need to empty your breasts regularly to avoid mastitis. If your baby is having surgery and cannot nurse, use an electric breast pump to draw off the milk, which can be given to her later.

If you have other children and cannot be with her all the time, try to arrange for another familiar person to be there when you are not. Night times are especially important; if you cannot stay, perhaps her father or grandmother can. They can give the baby your expressed milk.

You in hospital

This is a more difficult situation particularly if it is an emergency. Adult wards do not usually have facilities for mothers to look after their babies, unless you have a private room and the permission of the doctors and nursing staff. Other ways of keeping in contact with your baby include: for her father or babysitter to bring her to the hospital twice (or more) a day for you to feed her; for you to have outpatients' treatment or a very short stay with the rest of your nursing care at home (depending on your illness); for your treatment to be postponed until the baby is partially or totally weaned (depending on her age); or, very exceptionally, for the baby to be kept in the paediatric ward and brought to you for feeding (though she may be happier with familiar faces at home; the risk of infection is also greater for her in hospital).

Whatever you do, your breasts need to be emptied, and your baby should not be abruptly weaned if it can be avoided. If you can't nurse the baby regularly, you will need an electric pump to draw off the milk and your partner or visitors can take the milk home for the baby.

If your treatment involves strong drugs, you will need to discuss feeding with your doctor. For most conditions there is a drug that is suitable for nursing mothers; few conditions require the baby to be weaned only because of the mother's medication.

Wet nursing

If you are rushed into hospital in an emergency and your baby has to have breast milk (for example if she is allergic to other kinds of milk), you could arrange for another nursing mother to feed her. Babies can be successfully breastfed by women other than their mothers and these women can produce enough milk to sustain more than one baby so long as the extra sucking stimulus is there.

Some mothers babysit for each other and nurse each other's babies. This is much easier than expressing or preparing bottles. You may find that some people disapprove of this though there is no reason why they should. Until the end of the last century, wet nursing was an honourable profession and in many third-world countries it is still the safest form of substitute mothering.

Relactating

If you have produced milk, and then stopped for a while, it is possible to start again by building up the stimulus to the breasts from the baby's sucking. The ease and success of relactation will depend upon how recently you gave up breastfeeding and how much you want to re-establish it.

You need to nurse the baby every two hours or so – or as often as you can manage. She will need to continue with the formula and it may take time for her to learn or relearn the sucking technique of breastfeeding, so be patient. The best device for helping relactating mothers is the Lact-Aid. This enables the baby to receive her formula at the same time as she is sucking at the breast. Thus she is encouraged to stimulate the breast; she is getting fed; she is using the proper sucking technique; and you are both getting emotional satisfaction and physical closeness from nursing.

Reducing formula feeds

You should discuss your use of the Lact-Aid with your doctor so that you know the amounts your baby should be getting. Signs that you can start reducing the amount of formula are tingling, leaking and fullness in your breasts, the baby going longer between feeds and leaving some supplement in the Lact-Aid bag, and softer bowel movements.

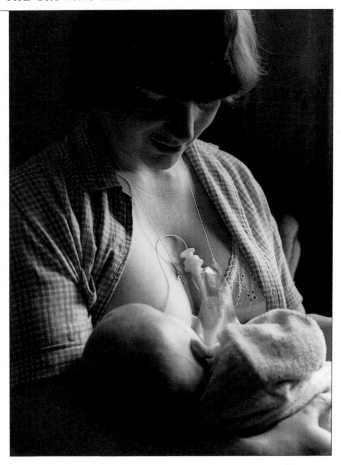

The Lact-Aid bag, filled with formula feed, is worn around the mother's neck and the fine tube is placed against the nipple. The baby sucks on both tube and nipple, thereby receiving the formula feed and stimulating the mother's supply at the same time.

You must reduce the supplements gradually; you could use a similar system to that on page 67, but for relactation, the reduction will need to be spread over several weeks. You may not succeed in completely breastfeeding your baby but if you both enjoy nursing and the benefits of breast milk are important for your baby, even partial relactation is worth while.

Breastfeeding an adopted baby

If you have had a baby before, and thus produced milk, your chances of partially breastfeeding an adopted baby will be greater than if you have never given birth. The younger the baby, the easier it will be to establish lactation.

If you have never had a baby before, the baby's sucking can still trigger off the milk-producing process, though not so efficiently, and the whole process of establishing supply may take longer. Supplemented by the Lact-Aid, many women have produced some breast milk for their adopted babies and enjoyed the closeness of nursing.

8 WORKING AND TRAVELLING

It is often said that the breastfeeding mother is tied to the baby, but she is not tied to the house. The breastfeeding mother can go anywhere with her baby and never have to worry about feeding, or getting home in time for set meals. Modern, lightweight carrying equipment such as slings, baby carriers and buggies also contribute to this freedom.

Being carried around on his mother's back or front is interesting for the baby and allows him to see, and be seen by, the rest of the world. In the past few years, as breastfeeding has become more common among busy women, Western babies have begun to enjoy the privileges of babies in less-developed societies, that is being carried around by their mothers and being part of the community, instead of being banished to solitary cribs for hours.

It is easy to go out with a young baby who is light enough to be carried in a sling. Depending on your build and the strength of your back, you can carry him like this until he is a few months old. Once he weighs 5–6 kg (11–13 lb), this may become too tiring for you and a lightweight carrycot/pram and transporter or a lie-back buggy may be easier for a long outing or carrying him to and from your place of work and the baby's crèche or the person taking care of him. When he can sit up with your support, he can be carried in a rucksack-type carrier on your back.

If you travel by car often, a padded baby basket or cocoon with handles can be lifted in and out of the carrycot on the back seat and then the baby can be transferred out of this into his cot in the house. He should never be left to sleep unattended in his cocoon. He could roll over and suffocate. Babies can be carried around on public transport in these baskets while they are very small.

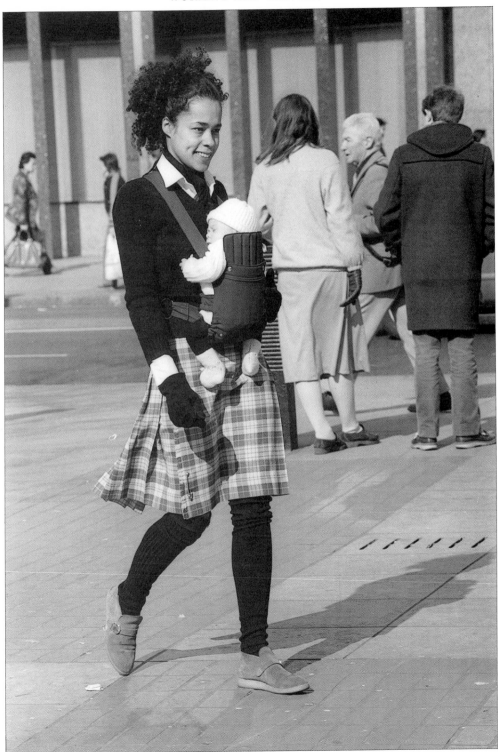

If you want to breastfeed when you are a passenger in the car, get in the back with the baby; never carry him on your lap in the front seat – the most dangerous seat in the car.

Working mothers

Many countries now have legal arrangements that protect women's jobs when they have a baby. Under such arrangements (which vary in generosity depending on where you live, what your job is, how long you have been employed in it and the strength of your trade union) an expectant mother is entitled to a number of weeks off work, before and after the birth, with some pay. If you are not sure what you are entitled to in your company, you should contact your personnel manager, trade union or professional representative and find out. You may be entitled to a longer period of leave, more money and less restrictive conditions than the government provides. Some employers provide paternity leave too, usually about two weeks at the time of the birth.

The decision to work

The decision to go back to work after you've had your baby is a difficult one to make; you do usually have to commit yourself when you are still pregnant. You cannot know how you are going to manage emotionally and financially, what sort of baby you are going to have and how you are going to feel about the baby – whether you are going to fall overwhelmingly in love with him or whether he's going to be difficult and irritating. If you intend to breastfeed, one thing you do know is that your baby is going to need you around for at least the first four to six months – so ideally your maternity leave should last this long. Some mothers return to work before this and breastfeed, but they usually have flexible jobs, either part-time, or local, or where it's possible to take the baby too.

The decision not to work

In practice, most mothers of pre-school children do not work, and those that do work part-time. This in part reflects the great difficulty most women have in finding substitute care for their babies. This is not a matter of the state providing crèches for everyone; it is a matter of you being sure that the person looking after your baby is someone you trust, that your baby likes and that you feel happy leaving the baby with. Such substitutes are rare; women who earn enough to pay for a nanny have a better chance of finding them. In Britain, registered childminders can be excellent mother-substitutes too. Many mothers simply feel happier looking after their babies themselves.

It is sensible to get your baby used to being with others though, such as grandparents, friends and neighbours, at first in your company and then for short periods alone. This gives you a break and it is also good for him because babies are sociable. If you can set up a system of visiting and babysitting with other mothers, you will all benefit.

Working and breastfeeding
Some practical points

If you do go back to work while your baby is still having an average of five feeds a day, you will need to do some planning. If you know you are going back to work when your baby is aged between two and five months, you will need to introduce him to his mother-substitute shortly after birth so that they can get used to each other.

Demand feed at the beginning to build up a good supply, but when the baby is about two months old, start to introduce a routine because you will need one to ensure predictability of feeding times. You will have to work this routine around the baby's natural waking and sleeping habits, but try to feed him as late as possible in the morning (say 6–7 am and then 8.30 am) so that the babysitter will only need to give him two feeds before you return at 5–6 pm. Breastfeed the baby before you go to sleep hopefully to avoid having to wake in the night. Working mothers often let their babies stay up later in the evening and encourage this wakeful time.

If you know that your baby will be having bottles when you go back to work, it's wise to get him used to sucking from a bottle early on. He can have drinks of water or diluted fruit juice from a few weeks old. This will not put him off the breast, so long as it is only about two or three times a week.

To ensure a good supply of breast milk while you are at work, you should express or collect milk for freezing at every opportunity, right from the start (see pages 72–73).

To make sure that you don't get engorged when the baby isn't emptying your breasts so often, you will probably need to express or pump while you are at work. Watch out for signs of blockages or mastitis (see pages 52–53) and take steps to prevent them. A pump is useful to carry with you as regular emptying of the breast also ensures that your supply is kept going. Many mothers work and continue breastfeeding for a year or more, more successfully than a lot of mothers who don't work. Surveys show that working is not a factor that stops women breastfeeding, so enjoy nursing and your job.

Working with the baby

Working at home

There are situations in which this might be possible and it obviously has advantages for the breastfeeding mother.

This is possible if you have a portable skill that can be exercised virtually anywhere (writing, crafts, bookkeeping, typing), although it will depend on the kind of work, whether you can find people willing to hire you, and whether you have the facilities at home to keep the work reasonably separate. If you have a placid baby, you may not need anyone else to mind him while you work. Once he becomes active and mobile though, he ought to have more attention. You can arrange things so that you work only when he is asleep, or in the evening. Otherwise you will probably find it less stressful to employ someone to come in and care for him for a few hours each day or for a few full days a week. He can still come to you for his feeds.

Taking the baby to work

A few places of employment have workplace crèches where children of employees can be looked after. This is obviously useful for the nursing mother (and many breast-feeding campaigners believe that there should be far more of them worldwide) so long as your employment conditions allow you time off to visit the crèche and breastfeed.

A workplace crèche enables a mother to continue breastfeeding her baby after she has returned to work. It also provides a way of introducing young children to breastfeeding naturally.

Some mothers have taken their young babies to work in shops, offices and schools while they were being breastfed. Once the baby is mobile though, a workplace without a crèche is not a suitable place for him. You also need to check whether your employer is insured for your child to be on the premises and, if not, that you accept full responsibility for him.

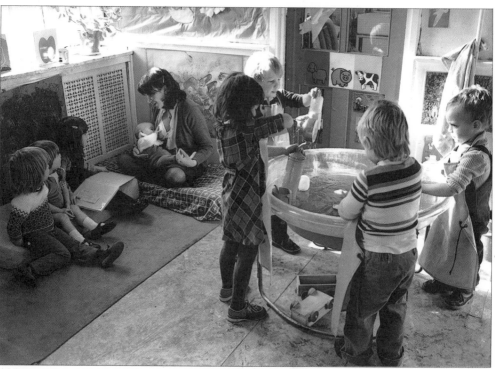

Breastfeeding while you are out

Some nursing mothers have happily breastfed in trains, subways, on park benches, crowded beaches, in restaurants, shops, museums, art galleries and in the street. The only comments they received were favourable ones – or, more commonly, nobody took any notice at all. Other women have had very different experiences of nursing in public: they have been arrested, turned out of public meetings, banished to lavatories, banned from restaurants and called offensive names for daring to breastfeed their babies outside their own homes.

It is difficult to know what might happen to you if you breastfeed in public; no matter how unembarrassed and discreet you are about it, you might just be unlucky enough to be sitting next to one of the people who make angry phone calls to television and radio stations when the word breastfeeding is mentioned on the air. In general, the more crowded and relaxed the place, such as the beach, the easier it will be.

Special facilities

Some shops and public places have special rooms where mothers can nurse and change their babies. If not, they may be willing to provide you with somewhere, such as an empty office, or a changing cubicle. Some breastfeeding organizations (see page 125) have lists of places which cater for nursing mothers; you may also get this information from tourist offices, local radio stations and from transport authorities. If you are planning a long expedition, it is worth telephoning these authorities and asking if there are facilities for nursing mothers and babies in their area. The more people ask for such facilities, the more acceptable and common the practice of breastfeeding a baby, in public if necessary, will become.

Planning feeds

It is a good idea to give your baby a feed just before you go out and to plan where and when you will give him his next feed. It's better not to wait until he demands it at full cry, as this will disturb you and make it more difficult for you to find somewhere to feed and to be relaxed about it. If you are going to a shop where you know there is a facility for nursing mothers, plan to be there about half an hour before you think your baby might next want feeding and feed him then.

What to wear for discreet nursing

If you cannot find anywhere specially set aside to nurse your baby, the best thing to do is to find a quiet seat somewhere, or go into a park if the weather is good, and feed the baby discreetly. This is easy if you wear the right clothes: an ordinary bra is probably better than one that needs a lot of hooking or unhooking, it can just be pulled up; in case of leaking, loose, dark or patterned clothing hides it better; a

T-shirt or sweater that pulls up from the waist is more convenient, you can tuck the baby underneath it; a poncho, shawl or loose cape can cover you both (so long as you are used to dealing with them); and on the beach, a large towel or beach robe serves the same function. Don't wear too many layers or belts and scarves that need to be unfastened; the baby may get lost inside them and he may lose the breast and panic.

These general guidelines apply wherever you are, for example if you are visiting friends or if friends visit you. It is possible to breastfeed without anyone knowing about it. The only thing that might give you away is the baby's noise: some babies are enthusiastic gurglers and the older baby can look on feeding time as a time for play (see page 106). Don't worry and try to quieten the baby, just respond calmly; even if those around you do realize you are breastfeeding, they are likely to take their cue from your matter-of-fact behaviour and not react at all.

Travelling and holidays

When you are travelling any distance with your baby and staying away from home, breastfeeding is extremely convenient and easy for all sorts of reasons. It saves a great deal of anxiety about carrying made-up formula and boiled water, about keeping formula cool and then warming it up, and about whether the water is drinkable or not. A fretful baby, tired from a long journey, can easily be comforted by the breast. Some mothers think they need to wean the baby before they go on holiday but nothing could be further from the truth. It is the worst time to wean, not least because you are introducing too many changes into the baby's life all at once; he may repay you by behaving awkwardly and your holiday will be spoiled.

If your baby is less than six months old, he can manage on breast milk alone while you are travelling. You can easily boost your supply (see pages 52–55) to meet the extra needs he will have if he has started having a little solid food, perhaps with his lunchtime breastfeed. If he is more than six months old and beginning to join in the family meals, he can have what you eat, thoroughly mashed up. For example, if you are in a restaurant, he can have a little mashed-up vegetable from someone else's plate, plus his breastfeed of course. If you have your own picnic food, or are buying food *en route*, he can have pear cut up and then mashed and a crust to chew. If you are travelling in a particularly hot country, avoid ice cream and cold meats. When eating out, give him only cooked food and fruit that has to be peeled.

Cans, jars and packets

If you're not sure about being able to buy food on your journey, some jars or cans of baby food are useful if the baby is used to having solids regularly. The packets of dried food are also useful, provided you have access to boiled water. (Your baby should have only water that has been previously boiled and then allowed to cool.) These commercially prepared baby foods are nutritionally adequate but they don't really taste very much like normal food. A banana mashed quickly with a fork or a miniature sandwich of wholemeal bread is just as 'convenient' on a journey.

Useful hints for travelling

It is a good idea to have a bag, with compartments, containing everything you might need for the baby in it. It is also wise to carry an extra disposable nappy, some tissues and baby wipes in your handbag, just in case you are separated from the baby's equipment bag.

If you are travelling by car and have a cassette recorder, cassettes of nursery rhymes and children's songs can be entertaining for a baby on a long journey and for the older children too. Their animation will amuse and divert the baby, with luck, preventing grumbles and crying. Remember that babies and young children should always travel in the back seat of the car in an approved seat or harness.

Is the baby having a breastfeed or just a cuddle? It needn't be difficult or embarrassing to breastfeed in public.

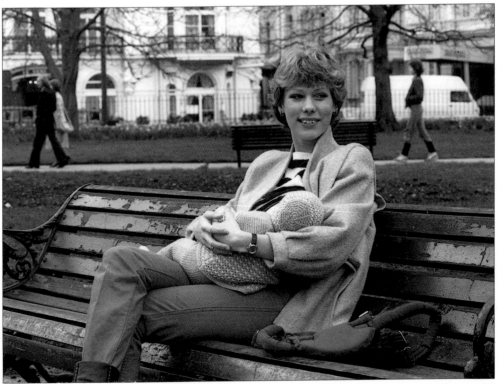

9
WEANING

In terms of feeding, weaning means changing from the breast (or bottle) to some other form of nourishment. Ideally the decision to make the change should be a mutual one between mother and baby. Some mothers leave the decision entirely up to the baby, but if you want to wean your baby completely from the breast at a specified time, you can encourage her to co-operate with you if you introduce the changes sensitively and gradually.

It is easier to wean a baby from the breast before she is one year old. After this she develops a will of her own and may resist being weaned. Many toddlers reach the stage where they 'demand' the breast in words. If you are happy to continue and see what happens, be prepared for the baby to do this. On the other hand, you may find that *you* are prepared to continue for 18 months or more, but she loses interest and decides to stop. As the baby finds other forms of enjoyment, nursing becomes less attractive to her.

Why other foods?

The nutritional components of breast milk and the amounts that the mother can produce are adequate for the baby until around six months (see page 28). This is only an average of course. In the weeks before this time, some signs may indicate to you that solids can be introduced.

Signs of readiness for new foods

If the baby is content and thriving, but at some time between four and six months she shows interest in other people's food, putting it in her mouth and chewing, then she may be ready for small tastes of solids. This is not an urgent nutritional requirement, simply a new experience. If she rejects the spoon and some of the new tastes, there is no need to worry; leave it for a week or so and try again.

If your baby is settled but then suddenly starts demanding

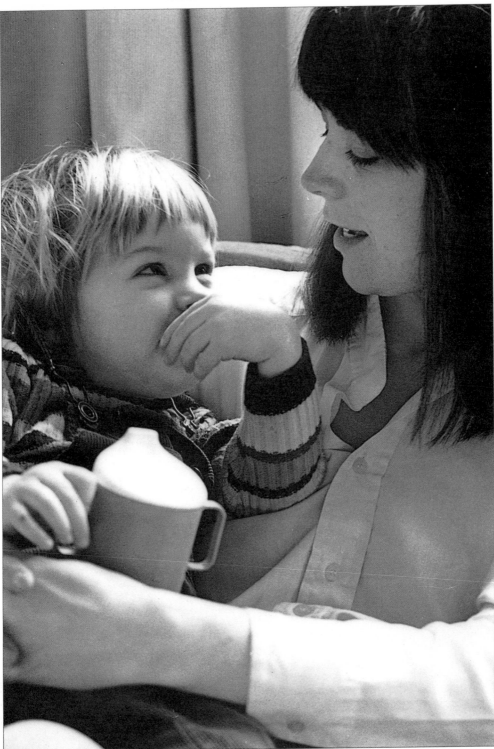

more feeds and even wakes in the night, this could be a sign for solids if she is over four months. If her weight gain slows right down, or even stops, and she was only average weight for her age, then she probably needs extra food. However, if there is no desire or need to begin to wean, don't be pressured by others saying 'Hasn't she started solids yet?'

Weaning to the bottle

Sample chart for rapid weaning: you can introduce the formula feeds at any time between the specified days. From day 14 onwards, offer the breast once a day until the baby is ready to drop the final feed.

Day	Breast-feeds	Formula feeds
1	5	1
3–4	4	2
5–6	3	3
8–9	2	4
11–12	1	5
14	1	5

What sort of milk?

Some mothers, including those who are returning to full-time work, decide in advance that they want to breastfeed for only three or six months and they stick to this decision. If your baby is still getting most of her nourishment from your milk, you must wean her gradually onto formula because, if you stop breastfeeding her overnight and substitute the bottle, you will become painfully engorged. It can also be extremely distressing and bewildering for the baby. Sometimes mothers who are having breastfeeding problems are advised to change to the bottle by their doctors, who should also give advice on how to wean at the same time.

If you are weaning to the bottle because you have been told that your milk supply is inadequate, theoretically you should have no problem with breast fullness and engorgement. In practice, many mothers in this position find themselves painfully dripping with milk. If this is your experience, keep nursing the baby at the breast, even if she has complementary bottles. There is never any need to stop breastfeeding altogether if you don't want to.

Start by dropping the breastfeed at which you have the least milk – perhaps in the early evening – and substitute a bottle of medically approved formula. You may like to follow the sample plan on the left. If at any time your breasts feel uncomfortably full, slow down the change-over. When the baby is down to one breastfeed, you may need to nurse her once a day for a week or two to ensure that there is no uncomfortable build-up of milk. Don't express when you are weaning, as this only stimulates your supply.

If you wean to a bottle when your baby is already having some solid foods, your milk supply will be less anyway and the change-over can be accomplished more easily.

Babies under six months and, some doctors say, under one year should be given non-human milk only in a modified form as one of the baby milk formulas. The majority of these are based on cows' milk and one formula is probably as good as another; be guided by your doctor's advice.

Many babies are allergic to cows' milk formula (see page 10) and ideally they should be given only breast milk for three months and preferably longer. If allergies run in the family, take expert dietary and medical advice if you need a substitute formula; don't just buy soya or goats' milk formulas as some babies are allergic to these too.

Once your baby is over six months, ordinary pasteurized milk is all right for her, as long as it is fresh and refrigerated. If you want to be cautious, boil the milk and cool it before you give it to her. If she has been totally breastfed for six months, there isn't much point in weaning her onto formula now. By this age you can avoid giving the baby bottles altogether, if you are still breastfeeding, by giving her all other drinks in a cup.

How to introduce solid foods You should drop breastfeeds much more gradually when they are being replaced by solids than when they are replaced by milk from a bottle. Your baby still needs primarily milk and plenty of fluids. Too many solids, too quickly, may be dangerous if the baby becomes dehydrated. The change-over may take about two or three months with the last comfort breastfeed continuing for a while after this.

Many mothers start by giving their babies cereal. Certain babies (coeliac-disease babies) are allergic to wheat-based foods because they contain gluten and many doctors recommend not giving anything with wheat in it to any baby for the first six months. It is easy to buy cereals containing rice or other grains; check the label for contents.

A toddler can still find comfort and refreshment at the breast when he is tired and thirsty.

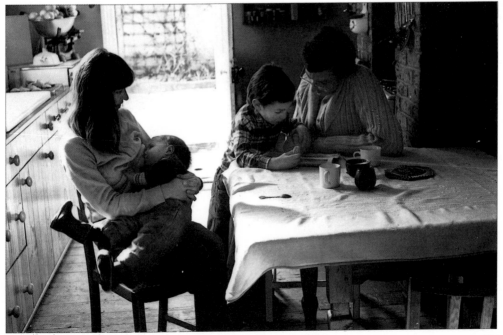

Problems with weaning

Problem	Symptoms	Causes
Baby's reluctance to be weaned	The baby insists on nursing for longer than you want, and asks for the breast at inconvenient moments. You feel resentful.	In her second year the child may be more determined about what she wants. You find it easier to give in. Other people may be putting pressure on you which is upsetting.
Mother's reluctance to wean	You may want to continue nursing but the baby seems to want to stop at around 6-8 months. She spits out the breast, bites, fusses and sucks only for a minute or two. May even refuse breast for comfort.	Some babies suddenly seem to get tired of breastfeeding. After the introduction of solids, your milk may diminish and the baby is not getting much. Feeding times are frustrating for her. Teething may cause her to bite.
Build-up of milk during weaning	Hard full breasts, pain in breasts, hot shivery feelings. You risk blocked ducts and mastitis because of engorgement.	Too rapid introduction of new foods. The baby suddenly loses interest.
Refusal of new feeding techniques	The baby refuses all other food except the breast.	Maybe you have started too early and the baby is not ready for new techniques. She may not like the taste of what you offer. Weaning may coincide with other changes and she may become suspicious of anything new.
The baby develops food fads	The baby refuses many kinds of foods including the 'good' ones such as fresh fruit and vegetables. She will only eat bananas, cereal, rusks etc.	Some foods are unpopular with many babies: eggs are an example. She may be an individualist with strong preferences.

First tastes from a spoon can be puréed fruit or vegetable. Commercial baby foods can be convenient but are also wasteful at this stage; offering her tastes from the family menu is the easiest and most enjoyable way to start. If she rejects any of these new foods try again at intervals of a few days, with different foods this time. As the baby gets used to an increasing variety of foods, you can give her one meal, perhaps at lunchtime, when her breastfeed is replaced by a drink of water or fruit juice from a cup.

Babies should not have added salt; it is not necessary and increases the risk of dehydration. Therefore do not add salt in the cooking. Babies should not have added sugar either, it is bad for their teeth. If they never have it, they won't miss it.

Solutions

If you have a really determined toddler you usually can't win in a battle of wills. Try to see continued nursing positively as convenient and pleasant. Distraction with other snacks, treats or a walk may divert the baby's attention and her desire to nurse. Seek the support of other long-term breastfeeders.

If the baby is quite happy with other food and drink, give in with good grace and enjoy her in other ways.

If your milk supply has diminished, there is little point in trying to build it up again at 6–8 months. If there is a special reason for her to have breast milk, such as allergy, try to build up your supply (see pages 52–55) if she will co-operate.

If she bites, remove her from the breast and say 'no' firmly. Watch her as she feeds, and when you sense that she is losing concentration, remove her from the nipple.

Give the breast first and slow down on the introduction of other foods.

If the baby won't nurse, you may need to express or pump.

Wait for a week or two until she has forgotten the insult and try again. It can take several tries before a baby accepts a spoon or cup. Don't get cross or she'll associate new foods with unpleasant experiences.

Try different tastes, there are bound to be some she likes. Talk to your doctor about a balanced diet based on these tastes.

Don't start to wean when moving house or when travelling; it is better to do it when the whole family is happy, relaxed and stable.

Babies will usually select a well-balanced diet if offered a choice. Give vitamin drops if she refuses fruit and vegetables.

Don't fight over it. Everyone gets upset and she still won't eat it. Check with your doctor to make sure that she is thriving.

Iron	After six months the baby's iron stores are used up and she will need new sources of iron. Therefore early solids should include iron-rich foods. Eggs may be an allergen, so if your family is allergic you may need to delay the introduction of eggs until later, when the baby is having an all-round diet. Other possible allergens are cows' milk products, nuts and fruits that contain pips. If you are worried about allergy, seek the advice of a doctor or dietitian; they can help you devise a well-balanced diet for your baby, based on foods she can tolerate.
Vitamins	These can be obtained from fresh fruit and vegetables; if your baby isn't interested in such foods, give her special vitamin supplements or drinks of unsweetened fruit juices

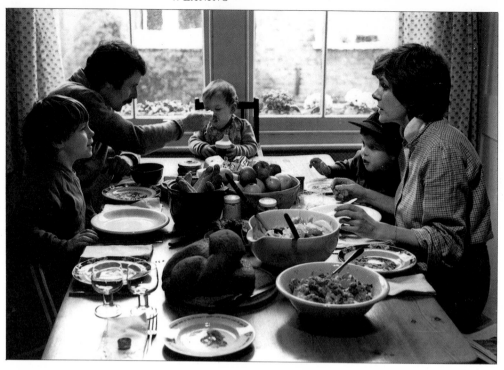

The baby is now part of the sociable world of the family mealtime.

Family meals

fortified with vitamins – there are special proprietary brands for babies in the shops. If you have dark skin and live in a cold climate, you and your baby may go short of Vitamin D, which is absorbed from sunlight. A wise precaution would be for you both to take Vitamin D supplements.

Gradually your baby will get most of her nourishment at mealtimes, just like the rest of the family. As she learns to bite and chew more efficiently, she will be able to cope with rusks and crusts and chopped-up meat, vegetables and fruit. As she becomes more skilled with her hands, she will learn to pick up tiny bits of food and crumbs and transfer them delicately to her mouth. She will learn to wield a spoon and get some of the food into her mouth this way. She will learn to drink from a cup and she will develop her own likes and dislikes, but as long as you offer her a wide variety of different tastes, she will usually select a reasonably balanced diet for herself. Nursing will become just a pleasant drink after meals and eventually the occasional comfort suck. One day she will fall asleep while playing and miss her goodnight feed and the next night she will forget to ask for it. Weaning in this way is thus not depriving the child of something she wants; it is a gentle process of substituting more grown-up pleasures for the childish pleasure of nursing.

RESOURCES

Breastfeeding and childbirth education groups
National Childbirth Trust, 9 Queensborough Terrace, London W2 3TB, England
La Leche League International, 9616 Minneapolis Ave, Franklin Park, Ill. 60131 USA
La Leche League Great Britain, PO Box BM 3424, London WC1V 6XX, England
La Leche League New Zealand, PO Box 2307, Christchurch, New Zealand
Nursing Mothers' Assoc. of Australia, PO Box 230, Hawthorne, Victoria 3122, Australia
International Childbirth Education Assoc., PO Box 19852, Milwaukee, Wis. 53220 USA
Assoc. of Breastfeeding Mothers, 131 Mayow Rd, London SE26 4HZ, England
Assoc. for Improvement in Maternity Services, 21 Franklin Gardens, Hitchin, Herts, England

International breastfeeding promotion groups
International Baby Food Action Network, c/o War on Want, 467 Caledonian Rd, London N7 9BE, England,
or c/o INFACT, 1701 University Ave, SE, Minneapolis, Minn. 55414 USA

Caesarean births
C/SEC Inc., 23 Cedar St, Cambridge, Mass. 02140 USA
Caesarean Support Group, 42 Shelford Rd, Trumpington, Cambridge, England

Stillbirth
The Stillbirth and Perinatal Death Assoc., 37 Christchurch Hill, London NW3 1JY, England

Handicapped babies
The Downs Children Assoc., Quinborne Community Centre, Ridgacre Rd, Birmingham B2 2TW, England
Caring (for parents of Downs babies), PO Box 400, Milton, Wis. 98354 USA
Assoc. for Spina Bifida and Hydrocephalus, Tavistock House, Tavistock Square North, London WC1 9HT, England
MENCAP, Golden Lane, London EC1Y ORT, England

Children in hospital
National Assoc. for the Welfare of Children in Hospital, 7 Exton St, London SE1, England

Twin clubs
Twin Clubs Assoc., c/o J. Linney, 198 Woodham Lane, New Hall, Weybridge, Surrey, England
National Organization of Mothers of Twins Clubs Inc., 3402 Amberwood Lane, Rockville, Md 20853 USA

Postnatal depression
Parents Anonymous, 8 Manor Gardens, London N7, England
Assoc. for Postnatal Illness, 7 Gowan Ave, London SW6, England

Equipment
Nipple and breast shields, bottlefeeding equipment, nipple creams, disposable bra pads, small hand pumps and pacifiers; these are all available from pharmacies. If you have difficulty in purchasing any of these items, contact one of the breastfeeding organizations listed above and they will advise you of the nearest stockist or the name of the manufacturer.

Breast pumps
Egnell electric breast pump, available from R. Davies, Egnell Rental Ltd, 66 Farndale Rd, Eastfield, Knaresborough, North Yorkshire, England and the NCT.
Egnell, Inc., 412 Park Av, Cary, Ill. 60013 USA (Local rental depots will supply a list.)
Kaneson Expressing and Feeding bottle, Happy Family Products, 1252 S. La Cienega Blvd, Los Angeles, Calif. 90035 USA
Kimal Scientific Products, Kimal House, Uxbridge Rd, Hillingdon, Middx, England

Information on adoptive nursing and Lact-Aid
Lact-Aid, Box 6861, Denver, Col. 80206 USA
Anne Buckley, 14 Brookway, Grasscroft, Oldham, Lancashire, England
Jo Young, 20 Grasmere Rd, London N10 2DT, England

ACKNOWLEDGEMENTS

The publishers and the author would like to thank the following for allowing us to photograph their families for this book: Teresa Askew, Diana Buxton, Tina Clarfelt, Marianni Cockburn, Marianne Dormsjö, Alicia Durdos, Margaret Gaita, Elsa Godfrey, Toni Greig, Mary Holroyd, Fran Johnson, Charyn Jones, Terry Keeble, Anna Leroide, Christine Lowe, Elaine McCarthy, Linda Moore, Denise Muschamp, Yuil Patterson, Joanna Rack, Bernadette Scally, Caroline Schenk, Freida Thornhill, Valerie Wayte, Ginger Weatherley, Lucinda Zarb. Thanks also to Sue Finch and Jill Crowe at the Kingsway Nursery, London; Sister Baker and Miss Henschel at Kings College Hospital, London and Sister Gould at Whipps Cross Hospital, London.

REFERENCES

REFERENCES

Numerals in bold represent the page in the book on which this research is mentioned.

(11) Richards, M.P.M. and Dunn, J.B. 'Observations of the Developing Relationship between Mother and Baby in the Neonatal Period', in Schaffer, H.R. (Ed.) *Studies in Mother Infant Interaction* (Academic Press, London and New York 1977)
(11) Hall, B. 'Changing Composition of Human Milk and Early Development of Appetite Control', *The Lancet* No. 7910 1975
(14) Martin, J. and Monk, J. *Infant Feeding 1980* (OPCS, London 1982)
(20) Robinson, J.E. and Short, R.V. 'Changes in Breast Sensitivity at Puberty, during the Menstrual Cycle and at Parturition', *British Medical Journal* May 1977
(23) Weichert, Carol 'Prolactin Cycling and the Management of Breastfeeding Failure', in Barness, Lewis (Ed.) *Advances in Pediatrics* vol. 27 (Year Book Medical Pubs., Chicago 1980)
(27) Ebrahim, G.J. *Breastfeeding: the Biological Option* (The Macmillan Press Ltd, London 1978; Schocken, New York 1980)
(29) Widdowson, E. 'Vitamin D in Human Milk', *Nutrition and Food Science* May/June 1979
(40) Salariya, E., Easton, P. and Cater, J. 'Early and Often for Best Results', *Nursing Mirror* May 1979
(40) Martin, J. *ibid*
(42) Klaus, M. and Kennell, J. *Maternal-Infant Bonding* (Mosby, St. Louis 1977)
(42) Richards, M. 'The One-Day Old Deprived Child', *New Scientist* March 1974
(53) Whichelow, M.J. 'Breastfeeding in Cambridge, England: factors affecting the mother's milk supply', *Journal of Advanced Nursing* No. 4 1979
(61) Francis, D.E.M. and Smith, I. 'Breastfeeding Regime for the Treatment of Infants with Phenylketonuria', in Bateman, E.C. (Ed.) *Applied Nutrition I* (John Libbey, London 1981)
(70) Gopalan, C. and Belavady, B. 'Nutrition and Lactation', quoted by Jelliffe, E.F.P. in *Breastfeeding and the Mother*. Ciba Foundation Symposium 45, 1976
(71) Jakobsson, I. and Lindberg, T. 'Cows' Milk as a Cause of Infantile Colic in Breastfed Infants', *The Lancet* August 1978
(79) Martin, J. *ibid*
(84) Martin, J. *Infant Feeding 1975* (HMSO, London)
(86) Cauthery, P. 'The Psychosexual aspect of Breastfeeding'. Paper given at International Breastfeeding Week Conference, London 1979
(89) Dunn, J., Kendrick, C. and MacNamee, R. 'The Reaction of First-born Children to the Birth of a Sibling', *Journal of Child Psychology and Psychiatry* vol. 22 1981
(92) Jacobs, B.S. and Moss, H.A. 'Birth Order and Sex of Sibling as Determinants of Mother-Infant Interaction', *Child Development* vol. 50 1979
(95) Lyon, M.L., Chilver, G., White, D. and Woollett, A. 'Current Maternal Attitudes to Infant Feeding Methods', *Childcare, Health and Development* vol. 7 1981
(97) Masters, W. and Johnson, V. *The Human Sexual Response* (Little, Brown, Boston 1966)
(101) Gomez-Rogers, C. *et al.* 'Effect of the IUD and other Contraceptive Methods on Lactation'. Proceedings of the 8th International Conference of the IPPF in Santiago 1967. (International Planned Parenthood Federation, London 1967)
(102) Wood, C.B.S. and Walker-Smith, J.A. (Eds.) *MacKeith's Infant Feeding and Feeding Difficulties* (Churchill-Livingstone, Edinburgh 1981)
(107) Kaye, K. 'Towards the Origin of Dialogue', in Schaffer, H.R. *ibid*
(118) 'Present Day Practice in Infant Feeding'. Report on Child Nutrition by a Working Party of the Committee on Medical Aspects of Food Policy (HMSO, London 1980)

BIBLIOGRAPHY

Goldfarb, J. and Tibbetts, E. *Breastfeeding Handbook* (Enslow Pubs. New Jersey 1980; J. Libbey, London 1981)
Brewster, D.P. *You can Breastfeed your Baby* (Rodale Press, Philadelphia 1979)
Macfarlane, A. *The Psychology of Childbirth* (Fontana, London 1977; Harvard University Press, 1977)
Phillips, A. and Rakusen, J. (Eds.) *Our Bodies Ourselves. A Health Book by and for Women* (Touchstone Books, New York 1976; Allen Lane, London 1978)
Present Day Practice in Infant Feeding (HMSO, London 1981)
Richards, M. *Infancy: World of the Newborn* (Harper & Row, London and New York 1980)